Pregnancy

BYWORD BOOKS™

We strongly discourage self-medication. The reader is urged to read the printed instructions of drug companies as well as consult a physician before using any of the drugs mentioned in this book because new side-effects are recognized and dosage schedules are being constantly revised. It is possible that errors might have crept in despite our best efforts.

First published 2007
Reprinted 2008, 2010 (in a new format)

10 9 8 7 6 5 4 3 2 1

ISBN 10: 81-8193-030-4
ISBN 13: 978-81-8193-030-9

Published by
BYWORD BOOKS PRIVATE LIMITED
Virat Bhavan, Mukherjee Nagar Commercial Complex, Delhi 110009
email: bywordbooks@gmail.com
Website: www.bywordbooks.in

Printed at Replika Press Private Limited, Kundli 131028, India

DoctorNDTV Team

Parul Chopra
Yatish Jain
Surjeet Bisht
Neha Vij
Pankaj Matta

Dr Anurag Krishna
Dr Anuj Sharma
Dr Nazli Siddiqui
Dr Shirish Kumar
Dr Samiran Nundy

Consulting Editor

Dr B. Shakuntala Baliga, MD (AIIMS), FICOG
Senior Consultant Gynaecologist
Apollo Hospitals, Bangalore
Sagar Apollo Hospital, Bangalore

Experts

Dr Puneet Bedi
Consultant, Obstetrics and Gynaecology, Indraprastha Apollo Hospitals, New Delhi

Dr Lalita Bhadwar
Consultant, Gynaecologist, Indraprastha Apollo Hospitals, New Delhi

Dr Punita Bhardwaj
Gynaecologist, Sir Ganga Ram Hospital, New Delhi

Dr Geeta Chadha
Senior Consultant, Obstetrics and Gynaecology, Indraprastha Apollo Hospitals, New Delhi

Dr Chandra Gulhati
Editor, MIMS, New Delhi

Dr Indira N. Hinduja
Consultant Gynaecologist and Obstetrician, KEM Hospital, Mumbai

Dr Sadhna Kala
Senior Consultant, Gynaecologist, Moolchand Hospital, Delhi

Dr Ashok Khurana
Director, Genitourinary and Vascular Ultrasound, The Ultrasound Lab, New Delhi

Dr Abha Majumdar
Consultant IVF and Reproductive Medicine, Obstetrics and Gynaecology, Sir Ganga Ram Hospital, New Delhi

Dr Mini Sood
Professor of Obstetrics and Gynaecology, UCMS, Delhi

Dr Pushpa Chandra
Obstetrician and Gynaecologist, All India Institute of Medical Sciences, New Delhi

Dr Rekha Sharma
Chief Dietician, All India Institute of Medical Sciences, New Delhi

Dr Kamal Buckshee
Obstetrician and Gynaecologist, Indraprastha Apollo Hospitals, New Delhi

Ms Nutan L. Pandit
Chairperson, Natural Childbirth Centre, Delhi

Dr Reshma Pai
Obstetrician and Gynaecologist, Lilavati and Jaslok Hospitals, Mumbai

Dr J. J. Amy
Gynaecologist, University Hospital, Belgium

Preface

In April 2000 during a convivial Sunday lunch at the Roys we were discussing how information on health was sadly out of the reach of most people living in India. Unlike the situation in western countries, especially in the USA, where important newspapers such as the *New York Times* had a special and authoritative section devoted to health every Tuesday, no such information was accessible in India. The newspapers and major television channels at that time carried few health stories and consequently anyone who was sick had to rely on a paternalistic doctor for all his or her health information. The busy doctor was usually reluctant to answer a patient's queries in detail and was likely to be irritated by the 'troublesome' patient who asked for more information. The patient was also hesitant to ask too many questions, as this would waste the doctor's time.

Two events occurred which changed the doctor–patient relationship in this country. The first was the passage of the Consumer Protection Act, which brought the medical profession under its purview in 1995. This allowed patients to take doctors to court for what they or their relatives perceived to be malpractice. The dissatisfaction with medical care was often due to a lack of communication between the doctor and the patient or due to the unrealistic expectations of the patient. Outright malpractice was rare as reflected by the very few judgments given against doctors.

The second event was the arrival of health websites on the internet. These began appearing in large numbers, most of them with obviously commercial intent and blatantly promoted hospitals, doctors or drugs. It was not possible to distinguish whether or not the information they provided was reliable. Nevertheless, these websites became immensely popular and, in the year 2000, it was estimated that 40% of American households were accessing the net for health information. Unfortunately, these websites targeted largely a western audience and carried little information of relevance to Indian patients because our diseases, technology available and social conditions were so different.

At that lunch we decided to start a not-for-profit health website in India which would cater exclusively to Indians providing them reliable information which was appropriate to their social and economic circumstances and would be of an 'international' quality. All of the information provided would be completely free.

We first sent emails to a hundred or so of our friends and acquaintances, who were leaders in medicine in this country and abroad, inviting them to join our site called DoctorNDTV. We explained to them that their responsibilities would include writing short articles on common and rare Indian diseases in a standardized question–answer format, vetting the material that our in-house staff produced and answering queries that had been emailed to us. All of this they were expected to do without any remuneration. Surprisingly, more than ninety per cent of these experts agreed to join.

We recruited medical colleagues – Dr Anuj Sharma, a web-savvy clinical microbiologist; Dr Anurag Krishna, a paediatric surgeon; Dr Shirish Kumar, a clinical haematologist; and Dr Nazli Siddiqui, a family physician – as well as bright young people to work on content – Pooja Gupta, Vibha Baluja, Jaieta Nag, Parul Chopra, Neha Vij and Surjeet Bisht – and technical staff – Sankalp Singh, Yugant Khanna and Pankaj Matta. Of these Parul, Neha and Surjeet are still with us while the others have moved on.

DoctorNDTV.com was launched in November 2000 and in its first year attracted about 5000 page-views a month and about 10 queries a day (all of which were answered within 72 hours). It is now the leading Indian health website for the general public and attracts over 4 million page-views a month and has 290 experts from all over the world who answer about 120 queries a day (the answer rate at present is about 90% – overwhelmed as we are by the numbers). From these we archive daily about 5–7 of the most useful and interesting questions and answers so that they are more easily accessible.

To make these archived Q&As available (and affordable, thanks to a subsidy from NDTV) to a wider public – those without computers or those on the move – we thought we would organize Q&As into printed books on individual topics. After analysing the kind of questions we are sent we found that the most frequently asked ones have been on sex, pregnancy and child development; so we have started the series with books on these three subjects.

After reading the DoctorNDTV books we hope that the next time you visit your doctor you will be able to better understand what the doctor says, and ask the most relevant questions regarding what's the matter of concern with you, and how and when things might improve.

Samiran Nundy
Editor-in-Chief
DoctorNDTV.com

Introduction

The NDTV Book on Pregnancy is designed to help women understand what to do and expect when they are planning or going through a pregnancy. The simple question-and-answer format is designed to explain routine and special tests, common and uncommon symptoms, as well as the effects of medication, supplements, unsafe lifestyle practices and environmental pollutants on the mother and her developing baby.

This book should not be used as a substitute for physician advice and evaluation. Rather, the expectant mother could use this easy-reading compilation of FAQs as a basis for building a simple knowledge base to make visits to the obstetrician more productive and interactive. Rapid advances in technology, genetics, microbiology and pharmacology are constantly changing the practice of obstetrics. The reader is cautioned that evidence-based practices and expert opinion presented in this book will have to be modified with the passage of time.

It was a privilege to accept Dr Samiran Nundy's request to edit this informative NDTV text on pregnancy. I applaud the editorial staff of Doctor NDTV and the experts for their commitment to patient education. I wish the potential parents among the readers of this book all the joys of raising a healthy and happy family.

B. Shakuntala Baliga
Consulting Editor

Contents

List of questions

Maintaining a healthy pregnancy

Tests and safety

Insurance

Abnormal pregnancy

Abortion and miscarriage

High-risk pregnancy

Problems of the fetus

Placental abnormalities

Appendix

Maintaining a healthy pregnancy

- Female reproductive system
- Growth of the fetus
- Skin care during pregnancy
- Sex during pregnancy
- Travel during pregnancy
- Smoking and alcohol
- Rubella
- Tests during pregnancy
- Ultrasound in pregnancy

- Common anxieties
- Diet and nutrition
- Pollutants and their effects
- Immunization and investigations
- Illness and pregnancy
- Infections
- Metabolic disorders
- Medications
- Tests and safety
- Insurance

Female reproductive system

The female reproductive system consists of the external and internal genitalia. The external genital organs are visible outside the body and begin to mature when a girl reaches puberty. Fertilization and conception takes place in the internal genital organs. The uterus, fallopian tubes, ovaries and the vagina are the main structures of the female reproductive system. The organs of reproduction are the gonads, which are the ovaries in females and the testes in males. The ovaries produce female gametes or eggs whereas testes produce male gametes or sperm. Sexual reproduction starts with the fertilization of a female gamete by a male gamete.

Females are born with ovaries that have hundreds and thousands of eggs, which remain dormant until the first menstrual cycle that occurs during puberty. During this adolescence phase, the pituitary gland secretes hormones that stimulate the ovaries to produce female sex hormones, including oestrogen, which helps the female to develop into a sexually mature woman. Females also begin releasing eggs as part of a monthly period called the menstrual cycle. During ovulation, the ovary discharges a tiny egg that reaches the uterus through one of the fallopian tubes, once a month. Unless the egg is fertilized by a sperm, it dries up and is expelled from the uterus. Fertilization can occur if a man and a woman have sexual intercourse within four days of ovulation. When the male ejaculates semen and deposits it in the vagina, fertilization occurs. This small amount of semen contains about 200–300 million sperms. They 'swim' up from the vagina through the cervix and uterus to meet the egg in the fallopian tube. However, only one sperm is required to fertilize the egg.

What is the menstrual cycle?

The menstrual cycle is a process through which a woman's body gets ready for the possibility of pregnancy each month. A cycle is counted from the first day of the period (menstruation) to the first day of the next. An average cycle is of 28 days, but anywhere from 23–35 days is normal. The day the bleeding starts is counted as the first day of the cycle. The menstrual cycle is controlled by hormones released by the hypothalamus, the pituitary gland and ovaries.

The menstrual cycle has four stages:

1. ***Menstrual phase:*** When a women has her period, it means that the lining of the uterus is breaking down and being discharged from her body through the vagina over a period of days called the menstrual phase. Menstruation is the term given to the periodic discharge of blood,

tissue, fluid and mucus from the reproductive organs of sexually mature females. The flow usually lasts 3–6 days each month and is caused by a sudden reduction in the hormones – oestrogen and progesterone. Most of the time, the egg released every month will not be fertilized, so the lining that develops each month for the possibility of a fertilized egg is not required. Over a period of days, the blood vessels shrink and the uterus sheds the unnecessary lining, made up of a small amount of blood and tissue.

2. ***Preovulatory phase:*** Menstrual phase (the period) is followed by the preovulatory phase (before the egg cell is released). During this phase, the uterine lining thickens with an increase in the number of blood vessels. The lining of the uterus needs to prepare itself for the possibility of supporting a fertilized egg. An egg also ripens in one of the ovaries for ovulation.

3. ***Ovulation phase:*** The third phase is the ovulation phase which occurs at midcycle, which in a 28-day cycle would be day 14. Ovulation occurs approximately once a month near the midpoint of a woman's menstrual cycle. A mature egg is released from one of the ovaries during ovulation. Some women may have slight discomfort during ovulation usually described as a twinge or cramp in the lower abdomen or back. Most women have no sensation while they are ovulating. The egg lives for twelve to twenty-four hours in the fallopian tube after it has been released from the ovaries and then disintegrates if not fertilized. If fertilization takes place, the egg travels into the fallopian tube and then begins a 4–5-day journey to the uterus. The few days before, during and after ovulation are a woman's 'fertile period' – the time when she can become pregnant. Because the lengths of menstrual cycles vary, many women ovulate earlier or later than day 14 of the cycle. Stress and other conditions can sometimes cause a cycle to be shorter or longer.

4. ***Postovulatory phase:*** The egg simply disintegrates in the postovulatory phase if it is not fertilized, the endometrium continues to develop and the uterine glands secrete nutrient materials.

   If the egg is fertilized by a sperm, it forms a zygote which attaches itself to the uterine wall. Fertilization usually occurs when the egg is in the fallopian tube. If a woman conceives, her menstrual cycle will stop during the time that she is pregnant.

   In the absence of conception, the hormone levels tend to drop. Below a certain level of hormones, the uterine lining can no longer be maintained and it breaks down; menstruation begins, and the cycle is repeated.

How can you know your fertile period?

A woman is most fertile during the midcycle. Ovulation generally occurs 14 days before the start of the next period. To successfully conceive, it is best to have intercourse within the fertile period, which starts about 2–3 days before ovulation. Usually, the fertile period in a woman with a 28-day cycle, extends from day 11 to day 18.

It is important to keep a track of your periods. Mark the calendar on the day you get your period. It is counted as 'day 1'. Count each day till your next period. You may need to do this for 3–4 months to accurately assess the length and regularity of your cycle.

- If your cycles are very regular, you may be able to determine when you ovulate: in the average menstrual cycle, ovulation occurs 14 days before the menstrual period starts – or on day 14 of a 28-day cycle. So if you subtract 14 days from the length of your cycle, you will get an idea of when you ovulate.

  Use the online **'ovulation calculator'** in the pregnancy section of DoctorNDTV.com to determine the most likely date of your ovulation.

- If your cycles are not very regular, or you would like a more accurate picture of your ovulation then:
  - Track your temperature: One of the indications that ovulation has occurred is a slight increase in a woman's basal body temperature during ovulation. You can detect this 'thermal shift' by taking your temperature every morning at the same time before you get out of bed. If you chart your temperature each day for a few months, you will begin to see a pattern that will help you predict when you are about to ovulate. In most women, the temperature increases by about half a degree 1–2 days after ovulation.
  - Watch for changes in your cervical mucus. This method does not exactly pinpoint but gives you some indication of whether you are in a fertile period or not. As your body prepares to ovulate, it produces larger quantities of thin, clear cervical mucus, a substance that smoothes the way for the sperm to meet the egg. On your most fertile days, just before ovulation, the mucus will appear clear, stretchy and slippery. After ovulation, when your fertile days are over, the mucus usually becomes thicker and then gradually dries up.

Tips to help a woman conceive

Having regular menstrual cycles and being healthy increases the chances of conceiving a healthy baby and carrying the baby to full term. Basic health tips include:

- Eat a healthy diet
- Manage stress levels
- Exercise regularly
- Do not smoke
- Avoid alcohol
- Reduce coffee consumption

If you are under 35 and have had regular unprotected intercourse for 12 months, or 35 or older and have been trying to get pregnant for 6 months, then it is time to see the doctor for a fertility evaluation.

When can you come off the pill

If you have just come off the contraceptive pill and are ready to have a baby, be prepared for the fact that conception may not happen straight away. The hormones in the pill have been running and regulating your menstrual cycle, not your body. When you come off the pill it takes a little while for your body to regain its natural hormonal rhythm, which varies from one woman to another.

Month-wise growth of the fetus

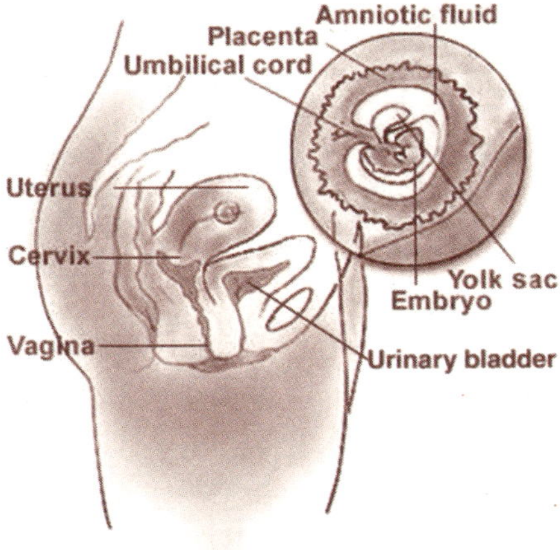

Month 1

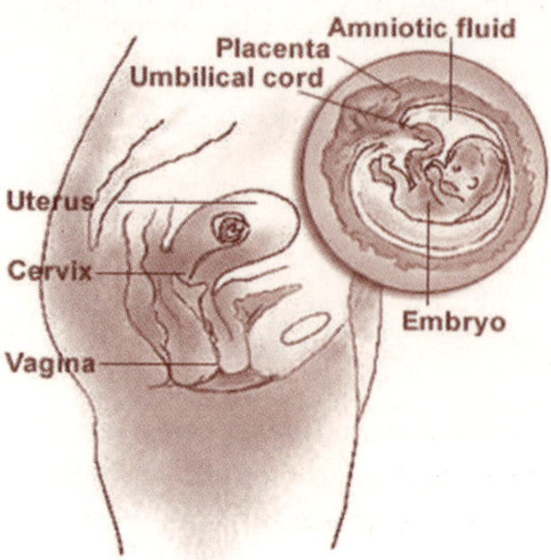

Month 2

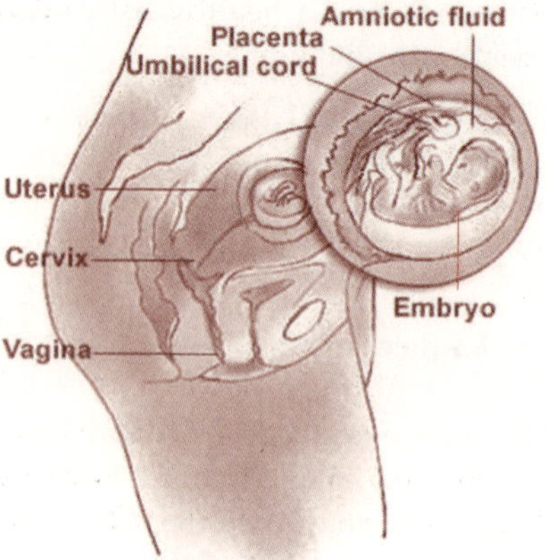

Month 3

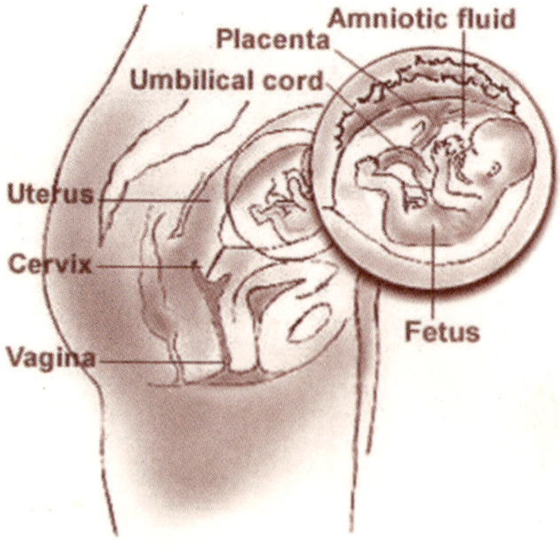

Month 4

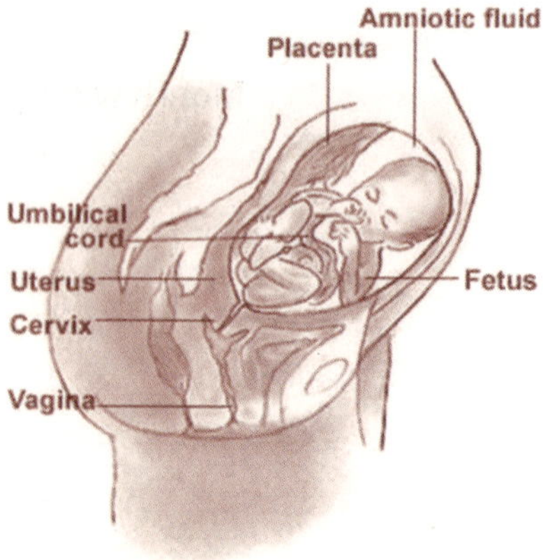

Month 5

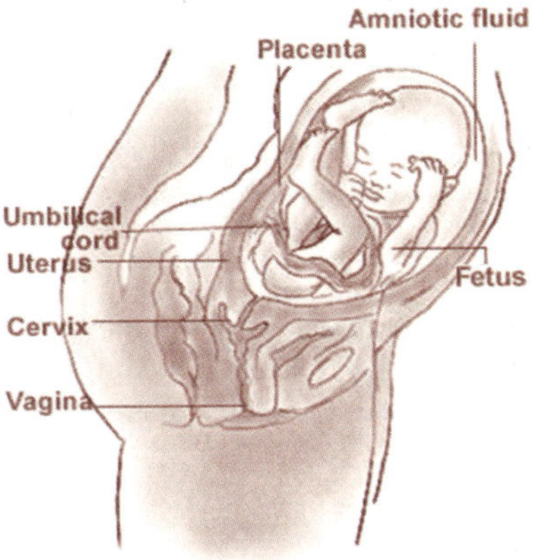

Month 6

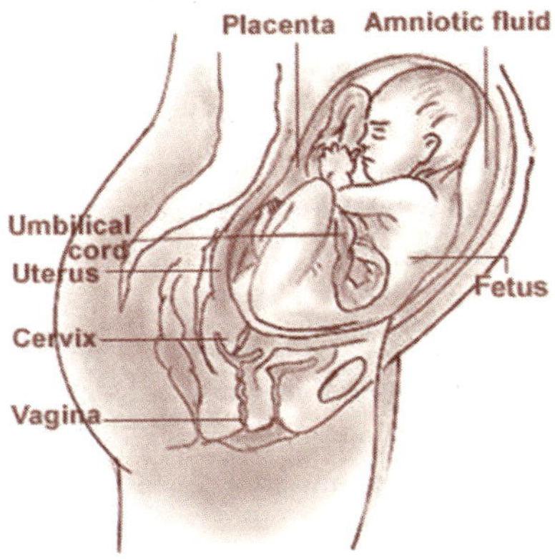

Month 7

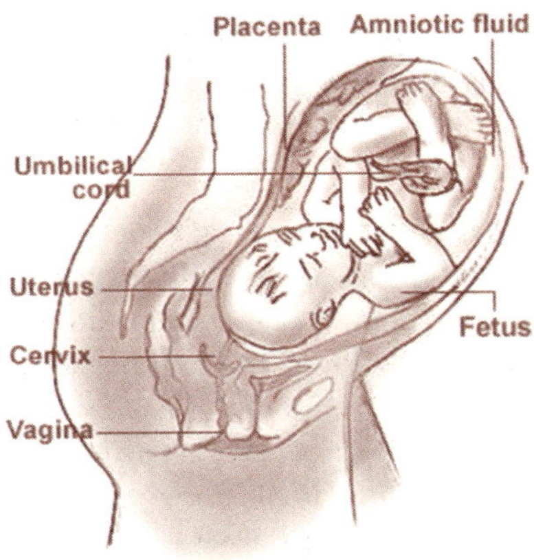

Month 8

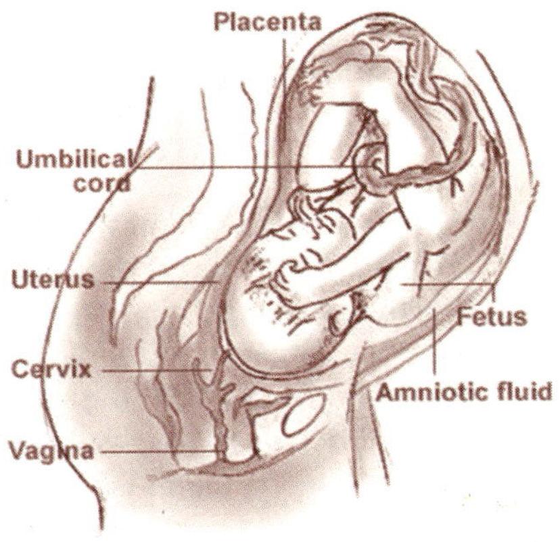

Month 9

Skin care during pregnancy

Pregnancy is a time of changes in the hormonal profile of the body, which may contribute to changes in the skin. Since the skin is the outermost layer of the body, even a slight change from the normal is evident. Pregnancy is also a time when special care should be taken to keep the skin healthy and glowing.

Many women frequently complain of dry skin due to overstretching but it is often taken as a normal part of pregnancy and no treatment is sought. However, some may also suffer from other skin conditions such as herpes, itchy rashes and mild discoloration.

Common skin conditions during pregnancy

- **Melasma or 'mask of pregnancy'** – It is a condition caused due to hormonal imbalance in the body during pregnancy. It is characterized by discoloration of the skin, mostly on the forehead, nose and the upper lip. The skin on these areas becomes darker in colour (looking like a tan) and may be wrinkly and may peel off easily.

  This condition may affect as many as 70% of all pregnant women, especially those with dark complexions. The condition is normally seen at the end of the second trimester or the beginning of the third. It does not have a specific treatment, but exposure to the sun makes it worse. Thus, women suffering from melasma should protect themselves against the sun by using potent sunscreens. In most cases, the marks vanish after the baby is born.

- **Urticaria of pregnancy** – Medically called puerperal urticaria of pregnancy (PUP), it is a condition of itchy rashes or hives that erupt usually in the third trimester of pregnancy. These rashes can be mildly or severely itchy, but usually disappear after delivery. Though they do not harm the mother or the baby, they are very irritating for the patient. Hives during pregnancy are usually soothed with ointments that provide relief. Calamine lotion is usually able to provide relief. Though drugs are usually not prescribed during pregnancy, anti-histamines may have to be given for itching in some cases.

- **Herpes gestationis** – Herpes infection during pregnancy is called herpes gestationis. It is characterized by the eruption of intensely itchy lesions on the skin that may be pus filled. This condition can occur at any time during the pregnancy but is most common during the second trimester. The rashes mostly begin on the abdomen and then spread to other parts of the body.

- **Acne and psoriasis** – Acne, in people who are prone to it, usually worsens during pregnancy. Psoriasis, on the other hand, tends to improve during pregnancy, but may flare up after delivery. Acne during pregnancy is usually ignored. Some drugs may be given to treat psoriasis, but they have to be taken only under a physician's supervision.
- **Varicose veins** – They are one of the most common complaints of pregnancy. Due to excess weight, most women develop varicose veins in their legs. Some may even have 'spider veins' on their face and chest. They usually vanish after delivery.

Tips for skin care

Apart from the medical conditions of the skin which may affect a pregnant woman and have to be medically treated, some basic skin care methods can be adopted that will help to maintain a healthy skin tone.

- **Sleep well** – A proper sleep pattern during pregnancy is one of the best ways to maintain a good and healthy skin. A well-rested person appears healthier and this is especially so when a woman is pregnant since she gets tired easily.
- **Sunscreen –** It should always be used before going out in the sun.
- **Clean the face thoroughly** – The face should be cleaned thoroughly since the skin of the face is usually oilier than the rest of the body. The pores of the face thus get clogged easily with dirt and cause pimples or acne. Cleaning the face regularly with a mild soap or face wash helps to prevent these conditions.
- **Moisturize often** – Since the skin is drier than usual during pregnancy, it helps to keep moisturizing it often. Women with oily skin could use a water-based moisturizer while those with dry skin can use an oil-based one. It is always necessary to follow a cleaning and moisturizing routine for healthy skin.
- **Get a facial massage** – Facial and body massage with mild and fragrant oils may be relaxing, apart from increasing blood circulation to the area.
- **Drink plenty of water** – The water balance of the body should be maintained. This also affects the tone of the skin. Water cleanses the skin and removes toxins from the body.
- **Smile and remain happy** – Happiness increases the blood flow inside the body and, thus, reflects in the form of a healthy and glowing skin.

Sex during pregnancy

Pregnancy is the time when most women experience a change in their hormonal profile to such a degree that they may have to alter a lot of their regular activities to suit their mood at that time. Sex is one of those activities which might be the most affected. Many women do not enjoy sex at all during their pregnancy while others obtain maximum pleasure.

Is it safe to have sex during pregnancy?
Sex during pregnancy is totally safe, if not advised otherwise by the doctor. Most women can have sex right until the last month of their pregnancy if they do not feel uncomfortable. It is safe to have intercourse since the baby is protected by a thick mucous plug that seals the cervix and guards against infection.

Some of the medical reasons which require abstaining from sex are:

- Recent vaginal bleeding
- Threatened abortion
- Preterm labour
- Ruptured membranes (broken water bag)
- Placenta praevia
- Infection with STIs

Does the sexual urge diminish during pregnancy?
Sexual urge is idiosyncratic and may increase or decrease when a woman is pregnant. Most women, however, feel a decreased urge to have sexual intercourse, which may be more due to the presence of other symptoms during pregnancy such as nausea and abdominal heaviness than due to actual decrease in sexual desire. Increased sexual desire may be due to increased blood flow to the pelvic area during pregnancy. There are changes in the hormonal profile also which may cause an increase in libido. Some women enjoy unrestrained sex since the fear of an unwanted pregnancy is removed.

The first trimester is usually the worst time for a woman to think about sex since most women experience breast tenderness and morning sickness during the first three months. They may also be tired both physically and emotionally due to the novelty of the situation.

By the second trimester the situation eases considerably and couples are more likely to resume their normal sexual relations. However, these preferences are purely individual and may vary from one couple to another.

By the third trimester, physical discomfort is usually increased to a large extent. This may prompt couples to adopt alternate sexual positions so that the discomfort is alleviated. The 'woman-on-top' position may be more suitable and enjoyable than the conventional 'man-on-top' one. The rear entry position or the side-by-side position may also be tried out.

Is oral sex safe?

Oral sex, especially during the later months, can be a very feasible alternative to intercourse. It may satisfy both partners without any potential discomfort. However, care should be taken that the male partner does not blow air into the vagina since it may cause blockage of a blood vessel which could be potentially dangerous. Oral sex should be avoided if either of the partners has a sexually transmitted disease.

Travel during pregnancy

Pregnancy is a time when utmost care should be taken of the pregnant woman's health, by herself and by others around her. Though travel is not prohibited during pregnancy, it should be undertaken with a few precautions so that the health of the mother and the child is not compromised.

The doctor may prohibit the mother-to-be from travelling during the first trimester since at that time the risk of miscarriage is the highest. Travelling may also have to be avoided in case of high-risk pregnancies or as advised by the doctor.

Is it safe to travel by air?
Most airlines have strict rules for pregnant travellers, wherein they are not permitted to travel if they are more than 32 weeks pregnant. Air travel may involve risk since the change in pressure may cause damage to the membranes of the uterus. Before embarking on a plane journey, the pregnant lady should take care to dress easily and follow the rules of the airline. It is better to not take the non-pressurized cabins in the aircraft since a change in pressure is dangerous.

What precautions should be taken during car travel?
Though travelling by car does not have any obvious disadvantages, long journeys may be avoided, especially during the first trimester. This is because the mother-to-be may not yet be used to the pregnancy and may get easily tired and fatigued.

Other tips to be kept in mind while travelling are:

- If the journey is long, frequent breaks (every hour preferably) are necessary to keep the circulation going in the body.
- If the seat belt has to be worn, it should be worn low on the hips and not on the abdomen to avoid undue pressure.
- Snacks should be carried on the journey to prevent nausea and to maintain energy levels in the body.
- A pillow should be carried to provide support in uncomfortable positions.
- The doctor should give a clearance for travel before the journey.
- In case of travel to a foreign country, the requisite immunizations should be taken well before the date of travel to avoid any complications.

Smoking and alcohol

Pregnancy is a time when the mother has to take utmost care to ensure good health for herself and her baby. Smoking, drug abuse and alcohol consumption are an absolute 'no' during pregnancy. During the first and last trimester, any of the above can cause irreparable damage to the baby.

How harmful is smoking during pregnancy?

Smoking at any time during pregnancy is dangerous, but is exceptionally so during the first trimester. Some of the conditions in the child that have been linked to maternal smoking are:

- Congenital heart abnormalities
- Small-for-date babies or premature birth
- Stillbirth
- Intellectual impairment
- Attention deficit, hyperactivity and behavioural disorders
- Learning disabilities
- SIDS (sudden infant death syndrome)
- MAS (meconium aspiration syndrome) where the newborn has a greenish, sticky liquid in his intestines due to inhalation of amniotic fluid during pregnancy.

Besides active smoking, even passive exposure to smoke is dangerous during pregnancy. The mother-to-be should therefore ensure that she is not even around people who smoke, as far as possible.

There has been recent evidence to show that the effects of maternal smoking during pregnancy are seen even after the child has grown up. Adolescent children of mothers who smoked during their pregnancies seem to have behavioural problems at school.

What is the effect of alcohol during pregnancy?

Pregnancy is unlikely to occur in women who are chronic alcoholics because of cessation of menstruation due to liver damage. Even modest consumption of alcohol (2–4 drinks per week) has been associated with miscarriage.

Alcohol consumption during pregnancy has many side-effects. There are many conditions that may affect the child because of consumption of alcohol by the mother when she is pregnant. The most common and dangerous condition is called fetal alcoholic syndrome (FAS). In this condition, the baby is born severely malformed and is usually mentally impaired. There may be defects in the heart, lungs and limbs. Children of about 10% of alcohol users develop this condition.

Other deforming conditions that may be caused due to heavy consumption of alcohol by pregnant women include:

- Increased susceptibility for ear infections
- Brain damage leading to mental retardation
- Low birth weight
- Difficulty in coordination
- Facial deformities

How much alcohol is safe?

There is no level of maternal alcohol consumption that is safe for the fetus. Ideally, alcohol should be totally abstained from, especially during the first trimester. If this is not possible, then the drinks should be reduced to less than 5 drinks per week.

Rubella

What are TORCH infections?

TORCH is an acronym for a special group of infections. These may be acquired by a woman during pregnancy, and include the following infections:

- Toxoplasma infection, also called toxoplasmosis, caused by *Toxoplasma gondii.*
- Other infections, such as hepatitis B, syphilis and chickenpox (caused by herpes zoster)
- Rubella, the virus that causes German measles
- Cytomegalovirus, or CMV
- Herpes simplex virus, the cause of genital herpes

What is rubella?

Rubella and measles are contagious viral infections, best known by the distinctive red rash that may appear on the skin of those who contract either of the illnesses. However, rubella is not as infectious and severe as measles, which is why it is also called three-day measles. But if a pregnant woman contracts rubella, especially during the first trimester, the virus can cause miscarriage, stillbirth or serious birth defects in the developing fetus – a condition known as congenital rubella syndrome. These defects can include deafness, growth retardation and heart problems.

What is the cause?

Rubella is caused by a virus that passes from person to person, hence spreading the disease. It can spread when an infected person coughs or sneezes, or by direct contact with an infected person's respiratory secretions, such as mucus. It can also be transmitted from a pregnant woman to her unborn child. A person with rubella is contagious from one week before the onset of the rash until about 1–2 weeks after the rash disappears.

What are the symptoms?

The signs and symptoms of rubella are mild and hard to notice, especially in children. The signs and symptoms generally appear between 2–3 weeks after the exposure to the virus. They last for about 2–3 days and may include:

- Mild fever
- Headache
- Stuffy or running nose
- Inflamed, red eyes

- Enlarged, tender lymph nodes at the base of the skull, back of the neck and behind the ears
- Pink rash that begins on the face, spreads to the trunk and then to the arms and legs, before disappearing in the same sequence
- Aching joints, especially in young women

How is it diagnosed?

The rash of rubella looks like many other viral rashes. Doctors usually confirm rubella with the help of laboratory tests. If the doctor suspects that the patient has rubella, he will do a virus culture or a blood test, which can detect the presence of different types of rubella antibodies in the blood. These antibodies indicate whether a person had a recent or past infection, or was vaccinated against rubella.

What is the treatment?

No treatment can shorten the course of rubella infection. Most of the time, the symptoms are so mild that treatment is not necessary. Doctors often recommend isolation from others - especially from pregnant women - during the infectious period.

If a woman contracts rubella while she is pregnant, she should discuss the risks to the baby with the doctor. If the woman wishes to continue with her pregnancy, she may be given antibodies called hyperimmune globulin that can help boost the immunity to fight the infection. This can reduce the symptoms but does not eliminate the possibility of the baby developing congenital rubella syndrome. Treatment for the congenital rubella syndrome varies depending on the extent of the infant's problems. Children with multiple complications may require early treatment from specialists.

How can care be taken at home?

In rare instances when a child or adult is infected with rubella, simple self-care measures are required:

- Rest is necessary.
- Take paracetamol to relieve discomfort from fever and aches.
- Tell friends, family and co-workers, especially pregnant women about the diagnosis, if they may have been exposed to the disease.
- Do not give aspirin to children who have a viral illness. Aspirin in children has been associated with Reye syndrome - a rare, but serious illness that can affect the blood, liver and brain of children given aspirin after a viral infection.

Can rubella be prevented?

The rubella vaccine is usually given as a combined measles–mumps–rubella (MMR) vaccination, which contains the safest and most effective form of each vaccine. Children should receive the MMR vaccine between 12 and 15 months of age, and again between 3 and 6 years of age - before starting school. It is particularly important that girls receive the vaccine to prevent rubella during future pregnancies.

Usually babies are protected from rubella for 6–8 months after birth because of the immunity passed on from their mothers. But if a child requires protection from rubella before 12 months of age - for example, for foreign travel - the vaccine can be given as early as 6 months of age. Children who are vaccinated early still need to be vaccinated at the recommended ages later.

Tests during pregnancy

Why does one need prenatal tests?

The woman's body undergoes considerable physiological changes during pregnancy that need to be monitored very carefully to ensure good maternal and child health. A pregnant woman needs regular medical advice to ensure that the pregnancy runs smoothly and any problem is detected and treated as early as possible.

What are the signs of pregnancy?

The first sign that most women notice is that their monthly periods do not start when expected. There may be other symptoms like nausea and vomiting. Some other non-specific symptoms that may indicate conception are:

- Frequent urination
- Tenderness and swelling in the breasts
- Cravings for certain food items like sweets
- Feeling of exhaustion or tiredness
- Backache

How can pregnancy be detected?

1. Home pregnancy tests are available as kits. Though they can be used to detect pregnancy fairly accurately, they should always be followed by a check up with the doctor. Home pregnancy tests work by detecting raised levels of the hormone hCG (human chorionic gonadotrophin) in the urine. In a pregnant woman, the concentration of this hormone increases in the body and is easily detected in the urine.

   To use a home pregnancy test, one must collect urine in a container and dip the test strip into it. Some tests are available in a plastic pad, and the urine drops have to be added to it. After waiting for some time (depending on the kind of test used), the results can be read according to the instructions given. Presently, only one test called 'Pregcolour' is available at chemist shops in India.

2. Blood tests – A suspected pregnancy can be confirmed with the help of a blood test which measures the amount of hCG in the blood and confirms the pregnancy. A blood test is more reliable than a urine test, so both are routinely done to confirm conception.

What tests should be done during pregnancy?

The various tests that are routinely done during pregnancy include:

- Blood group, haemoglobin and platelet count

- Blood tests for AIDS, hepatitis, rubella, and syphilis (VDRL)
- Ultrasound/sonography
- Urine test for albumin

Other tests may be required in special circumstances, particularly in high risk pregnancies. These include:

- Chorionic villus sampling (CVS)
- Amniocentesis
- Alpha-fetoprotein (AFP)
- Non-stress tests

Blood tests to diagnose Rh incompatibility (blood group of both hushand and wife), hepatitis, haemoglobin level and platelet count are done as a routine during pregnancy. An ELISA is nowadays also done to check for HIV infection. The specific blood tests are – Hb A2 (to detect thalassaemia carriers), HBsAg (to check for hepatitis B) and VDRL (for syphilis).

Ultrasound is a technique that uses sound waves to study the internal parts of the body. High-frequency sound waves (20,000 Hz and above), which are beyond the range of normal hearing, are transmitted to the area that needs to be studied and the returning echoes are recorded. The technical term for ultrasound testing and recording is sonography. It is used to listen to and monitor the fetal heartbeat and to check for any abnormalities in fetal development.

Conditions like Down syndrome cannot be diagnosed by an ultrasound, but certain abnormalities can be detected which may raise suspicion of Down syndrome. Abnormalities of the heart, digestive tract and kidneys can usually be detected in an ultrasound scan. Other conditions like spina bifida (spine anomaly) and placental abnormalities can also be detected.

Alpha-fetoprotein (AFP) is a test to determine the amount of a fetal protein in the mother's blood and the amniotic fluid. The amount of this protein helps to determine whether the fetus has any abnormalities. It is generally performed between the 15th and 18th weeks of pregnancy. Very high levels of AFP indicate an anomaly of the spinal cord. Low levels of AFP may indicate disorders like Down syndrome. However, the test is not totally reliable and has to be followed up by an ultrasound or amniocentesis.

Chorionic villus sampling (CVS) is a procedure in which a sample of the chorion (the membrane surrounding the baby) is taken for testing. The needle is inserted into the placenta but the amniotic sac is not disturbed. The test is used for checking for any genetic abnormality in the fetus. It is sometimes preferred to amniocentesis since it can be done earlier and the results are obtained sooner. CVS can be done as early as the 10th or 11th week and thus if any abnormality is detected, necessary steps can be taken almost 4–5 weeks sooner than with other procedures. The only disadvantage of CVS is that the rate of miscarriage is almost three times that of amniocentesis.

Amniocentesis is a test to check for any genetic abnormalities in the fetus and is usually done between the 15th and 17th weeks of gestation. A small amount of fluid from the amniotic sac is taken for testing. Since the needle is brought very close to the baby, this is done with utmost care under ultrasound guidance. The baby's position is marked very carefully before inserting the needle. An ultrasound is done to monitor the fetal heart rate, placental position and the amniotic fluid location.

Amniocentesis is advised for some women in the high-risk category. This includes women over the age of 35 years, women who have three or more miscarriages and women who have a family history of chromosomal abnormalities.

Non-stress tests are tests done to ensure the good health of the fetus without any invasive technique. The movement of the fetus in response to a sound or tactile stimulation is noted. There may be an increase in the heart rate or a sudden movement by the baby in response to the stimulus. The mother's abdomen is stroked gently and the response of the fetus is noted. If there is no response on repeated stimulation, then a stress test (invasive) may have to be done.

Ultrasound in pregnancy

Ultrasound is a technique that uses sound waves to study the internal parts of the body. High-frequency sound waves (20,000 Hz and above), which are beyond the range of normal hearing, are transmitted to the area that needs to be studied and the returning echoes are recorded. The technical term for ultrasound testing and recording is sonography. It is widely used in every branch of medicine and especially in gynaecology and obstetrics.

How is it done?

In this technique, reflection of high-frequency sound waves are used to produce an image of the baby inside the woman's womb. This allows evaluation of the baby, its organs, movements, etc. Ultrasound during pregnancy may be done by two routes – transabdominal and transvaginal. In the former, an instrument called a transducer is passed over the abdomen, while in the latter, the transducer is placed inside the vagina.

Is an ultrasound necessary?

Usually, two ultrasounds are recommended as a routine during pregnancy to monitor the baby's development. Some of the uses of an ultrasound during pregnancy are:

- To check whether the pregnancy is normal or complicated (ectopic pregnancy)
- To check whether there is a single baby or twins
- To make sure the position of the baby is normal
- To estimate the size and weight of the baby
- To check the position and attachment of the placenta
- To check the baby's heart rate and respiration
- To detect the amount of fluid in the amniotic sac
- To check for any fetal distress
- To determine whether the fetus has any physical abnormality such as abnormalities of the heart or kidneys.

An ultrasound to check for the growth of the baby is usually done in the second trimester (12–28 weeks), while that to check for the presence of more than one fetus is usually done between the 16th and 20th weeks. Though the sex of the baby can be determined after the 16th week of gestation, it is illegal to do so and can lead to fine and imprisonment. All ultrasound centres/clinics are legally required to announce prominently that sex determination is not done here.

Who should have an ultrasound done?

Though ultrasound is recommended in all pregnant women, it must be done especially in women who have a family history of complicated pregnancies, previous babies with abnormalities or those who have a gynaecological problem such as enlarged ovaries, pelvic infection, etc. The treating obstetrician usually determines when an ultrasound is required.

What preparation is needed?

No special preparation is needed for ultrasound scanning. However, it may be easier for the doctor to see the baby and its organs if the mother's urinary bladder is full. Thus, the mother may be asked to drink up to 6 glasses of water before the test and not urinate until after the ultrasound is over.

Is the test harmful?

Ultrasound scanning is usually not harmful for the mother or the fetus and is considered safe in pregnancy.

Common anxieties

1. Please advise me on good prenatal care during pregnancy.

Q. I tested positive in the pregnancy test. As this was an unplanned pregnancy, the news was a complete shock for me and I cried for the first two days. Will this affect the fetus in any way? I would like to overcome this and carry on, giving complete prenatal care to my baby. Please guide me as to what I should do for prenatal care, including diet/nutrition, exercise, thought processes, etc.

A. Congratulations on your pregnancy! It is good that you are looking forward to having the baby.

You must see your gynaecologist/obstetrician to schedule a complete physical examination. The first prenatal visit involves screening for many infections that have the potential for harming the baby. There is usually a screening for sexually transmitted diseases during the first visit.

Drink at least 4–5 cups of milk/equivalent milk products a day (the baby needs calcium to form its bones). The most important vitamin during pregnancy is folic acid. Walking is a good exercise during pregnancy. Lastly, you are fortunate to be pregnant during the internet era. You have access to a vast database on pregnancy, nutrition, etc. All the best!

2. What is the best age to conceive?

Q. We have been married for one-and-a-half years. I am 36 years old and my wife is 32 years. For the first 6 months, we used oral contraceptive pills and

condoms and after that, we haven't used any contraception. Since she did not conceive, I went for semen testing, which was normal. The details are: Volume: 1 ml, Reaction: alkaline, Colour: greyish white, Viscosity: viscous, Time of liquefaction: 38 min, pH: 7.4, Appearance: opaque fluid, Motility: 45% spermatozoa are actively motile, 20% spermatozoa are sluggishly motile, rest are non-motile, Total count: 70 million/ml, Fructose: 405 mg/ml, Morphology: smear shows 80%–90% normal spermatozoa. Now I have to take my wife to the doctor. She says she wants some more time (say another 4 months) in order to mentally prepare herself to meet the doctor. If I was 28 and my wife 24, we could have waited. But she is 32 now and by the time she becomes pregnant, I am worried her pregnancy may become complex. I don't know how to convince my wife.

A. The best time for women to conceive is before 30 years. This is important to have a healthy child. 32 years is still all right but after 35 years, the chances of conception start decreasing and the child could develop some anomalies. You need to address the fears she has in her mind. Your marriage should be stable and your relations with her should be reassuring for long-term happiness. She must spell out her fears frankly. As for the treatment, you must get her checked up and start with intrauterine insemination (IUI). IUI is the process by which semen collected from the husband by masturbation, is inserted into the uterus by the obstetrician using a special device.

3. Why am I not conceiving?

Q. I am a married woman with a 4-year-old child. We plan to have another baby but I am unable to conceive. I approached a gynaecologist who asked me to have the fallopian tubes checked for blockages by HSG/sonography. The result was normal and the tubes were clear without any blockages; the uterus was normal too. I was kept under watch through sonography for an ovulation check and it was found that ovulation took place on the 16th day. The doctor told me to make contact on that day but I am still not able to conceive. How can I conceive?

A. In general, if you have only been trying for less than a year, there is no need to worry. It usually takes up to one year to conceive. After that, some sort of work-up is in order. Do not stress yourself too much about days etc. Stress, in fact, interferes with your ability to conceive. Please talk to your doctor.

4. What is the best position to sleep in during pregnancy? Can I lift my daughter who weighs 12 kg?

Q. I am a 28-year-old woman with a 3-and-a-half-year-old daughter. I am planning a second child and want to find out what is the best position for me to lie down at night during pregnancy. Is it safe to lie on my back? Can I pick up my daughter (who weighs 12 kg) at night to take her to the toilet?

A. Any position of comfort is all right to sleep in except on your tummy; in the later part of pregnancy lying in the left lateral position is best for the baby, i.e. lie on your left side.

I would advise you to refrain from lifting your 3-year-old during pregnancy, as when you bend and then straighten to lift her up, you increase the abdominal pressure, which could start uterine contractions. The best way to lift any weight (should not be more than 8 kg) that one might need to is by first sitting with bent knees and then lifting, instead of bending and lifting. This reduces the strain on the back and is easier as well.

5. We are not very comfortable while having sex. Is this normal during pregnancy?

Q. I am 5 months pregnant. My husband and I face a lot of discomfort while having sex. Despite the fact that I have a lot of lubrication, it feels very tight, almost like he's touching my cervix. Is this normal?

A. Yes, due to the growing womb, the cervix does come down a bit. There is a lot more lubrication (and secretions) in the vaginal canal during pregnancy due to the influence of hormones. Both these events are normal. We suggest, if it is all right with both of you, that you try the sideways or the woman-on-top position instead of the conventional man-on-top position. Both of you will be more comfortable, as you shall be able to control the penetration much better.

However, vaginal sex is best avoided in women who have the cervical stitch, those on treatment for threatened abortion, those who have a history of preterm labour in the previous pregnancy, and those being treated for preterm labour, preterm leakage of 'water' and bleeding during pregnancy.

6. Will having sex during pregnancy lead to problems in delivery?

Q. **My wife is 24 years old. She is 7 months pregnant. We got married 10 months back. Till date we haven't had a full-fledged sexual intercourse. Even our occasional contacts are very infrequent, but somehow she conceived. Some of my friends say that sexual intercourse during pregnancy will make the delivery a bit complicated. Is it true that having more sex will result in widening the vagina and a case like ours will end up in a caesarean?**

A. No, there is no relation between sex during pregnancy and a difficult delivery. Similarly, having more sex during pregnancy doesn't result in widening of the vagina. Your friends are obviously ignorant of the facts. This is a situation where a blind person is leading another blind person!

7. Can I do abdominal exercises during pregnancy?

Q. **I wanted to know something regarding exercises and pregnancy. Are abdominal exercises a risk factor in pregnancy?**

A. If you have already been exercising before your pregnancy, then you may continue to do so, if your gynaecologist/obstetrician has given you the go-ahead. You would be better off doing reverse curls, which is to sit, with your knees slightly folded and feet flat on the ground ahead of you. Now very slowly, go downward towards the back just as much as is comfortable. Do this a couple of times and then hold for a period of 5 counts.

However, if you are planning to start a programme now, then do refrain from it. You can keep fit by walking and doing stretching exercises. And get to it after you deliver.

Women with hypertension, those with growth-restricted babies, threatened preterm labour, abortion, leakage of amniotic fluid (water), and twin pregnancy should not exercise actively during pregnancy. Some studies have shown that those who continue with regular aerobic exercises or running exercises have babies with slightly lower birth weight. An experienced physiotherapist should be consulted for appropriate exercises during and after pregnancy. (*See also* page 186)

8. Can I swim in the 5th month of pregnancy?

Q. **I am 21 weeks pregnant. Can I swim?**

A. Swimming is a non-weight bearing exercise and is better than weight bearing exercises during pregnancy. However, you should be careful to avoid slipping on a wet floor. You should swim in a swimming pool that is maintained according to recommended standards to avoid infection.

Make sure that you have had at least one check-up by your gynaecologist/obstetrician and that everything is normal.

9. I am pregnant and not able to eat anything due to severe nausea. What should I do?

Q. I am 23 years old. I am 16 weeks pregnant and this is my first pregnancy. I am in the 2nd trimester now. I had very bad nausea in the 1st trimester and now I feel a bit better. I was not able to take prenatal vitamins and folic acid due to nausea. Is it too late to take them now? I lost about 3 kg (7 pounds). My weight was 50 kg (110 pounds) earlier, but now it is only 47 kg (103 pounds). I have not been able to eat much as yet. I try as far as I can. Please advise.

A. Make sure not to restrict your diet during pregnancy. If you do, you might not take in the right amounts of protein, vitamins and minerals that are necessary to properly nourish your unborn baby. Folic acid helps prevent serious birth defects of your baby's brain and spine. Please see your doctor immediately so that he can start you on the suitable dose of vitamins and folic acid. Morning sickness and nausea are common problems in pregnant women. Most nausea occurs during the early part of pregnancy and, most likely, will subside now that you have entered the second trimester. The changes in your body might cause nausea or the urge to vomit when you smell or eat certain things, when you are tired or stressed, and sometimes for no apparent reason at all. Nausea in early pregnancy is a condition that often can be managed by changing when and what you eat.

Severe nausea and vomiting in pregnancy that continues beyond the first trimester is rare, but if it occurs, it can cause you to become dehydrated. If your nausea or vomiting is keeping you from eating right and has made you lose weight, talk with your doctor immediately.

Try these tips as well:

- Eat smaller and more frequent meals, such as six to eight small meals per day instead of three large ones.
- Avoid being without food for long periods of time.

- Drink plenty of fluids between, but not with, meals.
- Avoid greasy, fried or spicy food.
- Avoid foul and unpleasant odours that increase the feeling of nausea. For example, deodorants which you otherwise liked may make you nauseous during pregnancy. Avoid all strong smells.
- Rest when you are tired. Even if you are working, put your feet up on a chair when feeling tired, and sit back for a while.

In your case, the weight loss is significant. Other causes of persistent vomiting and weight loss need to be ruled out. Treatment with antiemetics, psychological support and parenteral (intravenous) nutrition may be required.

10. What are the causes of bleeding and spotting during pregnancy?

Q. What are the causes of and remedies for bleeding and spotting during pregnancy? Can it affect the baby if my wife gets pregnant next time?

A. The causes of bleeding and spotting during pregnancy are varied:

1st trimester

- Subchorionic haematomas: Complete bed rest is required.
- Luteal phase defects: Progesterone injections are given.
- Cervical erosion: Normal phenomenon during pregnancy; requires bed rest.

3rd trimester

- Placenta praevia (wherein the placenta is low lying): May lead to spotting or excessive bleeding; requires complete bed rest
- Placental abruption (wherein the placenta separates before the birth of the baby leading to heavy bleeding): Immediate intervention may be required to save the mother and fetus.
- Vasa praevia (wherein part of the placenta overlies the os and tearing of these vessels may cause severe bleeding): May require ceasarean section to save the fetus.

The chances of recurrence of bleeding are not very high in subsequent pregnancies. However, utmost care has to be taken; hormonal support may be required with complete bed rest from early pregnancy.

11. What causes vaginal discharge during pregnancy?

Q. My wife is pregnant. She had vaginal discharge 20 days before her due date, which lasted for three days and then stopped. She is also unable to sleep at night and has severe back pain. Kindly advise if there is a serious problem.

A. Vaginal discharge during pregnancy, especially full term pregnancy as in your case, should be immediately investigated because it could be a leakage of fluid around the baby, which, if left untreated, could cause infection in the baby.

Preterm rupture of the membranes (PROM, i.e. leakage of water) and vaginal infections need to be ruled out in this case. These conditions can be diagnosed only by an internal (vaginal) examination of your wife using a speculum. Please treat this as urgent as both conditions have deleterious effects on the baby, and should be treated immediately.

12. What is the cause for pain in the pubic area during pregnancy?

Q. I am 28 years old (height: 5'5", current weight: 69 kg). This is my first pregnancy and I am in my 7th month. For the past 2–3 days, I have been having pain in the labia majora and its vicinity, which is aggravated on walking and doing other chores. While resting or sitting or even touching the area, I feel no pain. It seems that I have no pain in the abdomen also. Till now I had no problem and I continue to work even though my haemoglobin is 8.9 g/dl.

A. You have not mentioned your latest blood pressure (BP) and whether or not you have swelling over the feet or on the labia majora. If your BP is normal and you do not have swelling over the feet and on the labia, this could be due to:

- Pain in the pubic bones and pain due to softening of the ligaments in the pubic area as a result of changes during pregnancy which is interpreted as pain in the area you have mentioned. Walking and doing other chores would obviously aggravate this pain. Be sure to take sufficient calcium in the form of milk and milk products supplemented by 1 g of elemental calcium per day (e.g. Ostocalcium tablet 500 mg twice daily).
- Local infection, which can be diagnosed by your obstetrician.

Your haemoglobin level is of concern. You must have complete blood counts done, including a peripheral smear, to diagnose the type and cause of anaemia. You must have your obstetrician correct your anaemia immediately, and she will be able to tell you whether or not you need to be screened for thalassaemia. A check-up by your obstetrician will clear all your doubts.

13. Why do I have abdominal pain during pregnancy?

Q. I went through the pregnancy test and the result was positive. I suffer from continuous abdominal pain, which my doctor says will be there to some extent. However, my pain is quite severe. I weigh 36 kg and am about 5 feet tall. Please advise. I generally suffer from pain at night. I do not understand why. Could you please help me out? How can we detect miscarriage, if so, in 7th to 9th week of pregnancy?

A. Pain in the abdomen is common in early pregnancy. It is due to the growing baby and the hormonal changes within the body during pregnancy. However, please visit your gynaecologist/obstetrician to rule out any other reason for the pain, which could harm continuation of the pregnancy. You are underweight for the height mentioned and must improve your dietary intake and thus the weight.

Symptoms of miscarriage are severe abdominal pain, bleeding and passing pieces of tissue through the vagina.

14. Will my back pain reappear after delivery?

Q. I am 28 years old. I had a fall 5 years back and was diagnosed to have disc prolapse at L4–5. I had backache with pain radiating to my left leg, and took bed rest for 6–8 weeks, did exercises and was absolutely pain-free till I conceived this year. My pain started again, radiating to my left leg, but was cured after taking bed rest for 8 weeks. I am 8 months pregnant now, but I fear that my back pain would reappear after normal labour. What do you recommend about the mode of delivery? How safe is lower segment caesarean section (LSCS) considering my history?

A. The exact relationship of backache and normal labour is difficult to predict. Whether normal labour will make the pain worse or better is not predictable. It depends, among other things, on what is the main cause of the backache. Disc is a common label but does not tell the whole story.

An orthopaedic surgeon or neurosurgeon needs to be consulted for this problem. If required, an MRI can be done to see the degree of disc prolapse. Accordingly, the treating surgeon will be able to advise you regarding mode of delivery.

Caesarean or CS is not a guarantee that you will not get backache, as the cause of weakened back muscles and ligaments is related to pregnancy hormones and not the event of labour. Needless to say, CS, if required for medical reasons and done properly, is safe these days. So please get an orthopaedic opinion and make a decision with the help of your obstetrician. It will not be easy to make a decision. But one cannot make a blanket statement that caesarean will ensure that backache will not come back or normal labour will essentially make the backache worse.

15. What is the cause for a surge in the resting pulse rate during pregnancy?

Q. I am 7 months pregnant. My routine check-ups with the doctor show that I have a regular pulse and blood pressure. But at least twice a day I find that when I am resting, my pulse goes up to 120 beats/minute. I want to know why this happens, what steps should I take and does this adversely affect the health of my baby?

A. You must get your sleeping pulse rate noted over 1 week. If it is high you must get thyroid tests done to rule out hyperthyroidism. However, it is interesting to note that your pulse is regular as noted by the obstetrician. Apprehension can lead to a high pulse rate, but that occurs when you are visiting the doctor, and not when you are resting. It is worthwhile being examined by a cardiologist for a complete evaluation of your cardiovascular system.

16. Is pigmentation of the skin common during pregnancy?

Q. I am 6 months pregnant. Since the 3rd month of my pregnancy, a straight dark line has been developing below and above the navel (stretching straight between the breasts right down to the vagina). Some people say it will disappear after giving birth but now at 6 months, it is somewhat thick and straight. Can you tell me what this actually is?

A. Hyperpigmentation (dark pigmentation) can be found in about 90% of pregnancies. Women with a darker complexion are more likely to manifest hyperpigmentation. The area around the nipples, umbilicus, and peri-anal skin may darken, and the linea alba (light white line between the mid stomach and pubic area) becomes the linea nigra (turns dark). Some women develop dark patches on the face. Most of these changes disappear after childbirth. It will be soothing for you if you protect your face from the sun or use sunscreen outside the house. (*See also* page 8)

17. Why does itchy rash occur during pregnancy?

Q. My wife is 27 years old, now 8 months and 10 days pregnant. Since the past 10 days, she has developed rashes around her stomach. Initially we thought them to be stretch marks, but later they started spreading fast across the body. It is a red rash and itches a lot. What is it? Is it some kind of allergy and what is the solution?

A. The itchy rash (if they are not stretch marks) on the abdomen of your pregnant wife could be due to

- Pregnancy itself: This usually resolves spontaneously after childbirth.
- One of the medicines she might be taking. Sometimes, it may even be due to preservatives etc. in the vitamin preparation, or
- Any other skin problem that can occur in a non-pregnant woman.

A clinical examination is necessary to differentiate between the above possibilities. The line of management would vary accordingly. Please contact your treating doctor for a check-up. (*See also* page 8)

18. Why do I have an itchy feeling during pregnancy?

Q. I am 3 months pregnant and the day before yesterday, I developed an itchy feeling all over my body. Some red rashes appeared on my neck which faded after some time. The same thing happened yesterday and this time the itching was worse. I do not want to take any medication in view of my pregnancy. What is this condition? Is it treatable?

A. From the symptoms that you have mentioned, it seems that you are suffering from a condition called urticaria. It is an allergic condition that may be caused due to many factors such as a drug or some food item.

I presume you have not been taking any medication, and this may be due to allergic reaction to a food item. To ascertain the exact cause, you must maintain a chart noting the time of occurrence of the rashes and what food item was consumed about 3–4 hours prior to the attack. You should also avoid high protein foods at this time.

Though drugs are usually not prescribed during pregnancy, you can take Avil (chlorpheniramine) tablets, which is a safe anti-allergic. However, you should not take any other drug, and even Avil must be taken under an obstetrician's supervision. For temporary relief, calamine lotion may be applied, but please ensure that it does not contain any anti-histamine. I suggest that you wait for a couple of days and if this does not subside on its own, you should consult your obstetrician.
(*See also* page 8)

19. When can one conceive after removing a copper-T?

Q. I am a 31-year-old mother of a 2-and-a-half-year-old child. I am using copper-T (Cu-T) as a contraceptive. We are now planning to have another child. What are the things to be taken care of while going for the removal of the Cu-T? How long do we have to wait for conception after removing the Cu-T? Will conceiving immediately be harmful to the fetus?

A. It is good to remove the Cu-T during the 3rd or 4th day of menses as the os (mouth of the uterus) is usually open at this time. There is no harm in conceiving the same month.

20. Is travelling recommended during pregnancy?

Q. I have to travel by road to high altitude (Kashmir) during the 5th–6th week of my pregnancy for eight hours. Should I accompany my husband on this trip?

A. Travelling – especially by road where the ride can be bumpy, at high altitude in Kashmir – is not recommended during the first trimester of pregnancy. Otherwise, travel by a healthy woman has no harmful effect on pregnancy.

The greatest risk with travel in your case is of a complication (e.g. bleeding) occurring away from health facilities required to adequately manage the emergency. Also, if nausea has already started, travel to a hilly area, at high altitude, can worsen the maternal condition. (*See also* page 12)

21. Should I continue with my job during pregnancy?

Q. I am 2 months pregnant. I recently took up a job but the place is 30 km away from my home. The first day in office was fine but while travelling in the bus, I felt nauseous and very uncomfortable. Would you recommend that I continue with the job?

A. Nausea is very common in the first 12 weeks of pregnancy. If you already have some disposition to travel sickness, the nausea will be worse. There is some evidence that ginger root helps. Taking it in the form of ginger tea before travelling may help. Whether to work or not is a decision you have to make for yourself, taking into consideration the availability of jobs, family support after the baby is born, etc. Good luck with the baby!

22. Do negative thoughts influence the fetus?

Q. I am 24 years old and 5 months pregnant. Will my present emotions affect the personality of the baby once it is born? For instance, if I am always anxious about something or if I am worried about a particular incident – would this affect the baby? I ask this question because many people say that negative thinking during pregnancy can adversely affect the child. Do our thoughts influence the fetus?

A. Scientifically, your emotions do not have a bearing on the personality of your unborn child. However, if you have negative feelings or depression, it can adversely affect your health. This, in turn, will affect the well-being of your unborn baby. The mantra for a good outcome is to be happy and positive in your outlook.

23. I conceived through IVF; will my thoughts and lifestyle affect my baby's personality?

Q. I have recently conceived through an IVF procedure and I am in my 4th month of pregnancy. I had a problem of polycystic ovarian syndrome (PCOS) and hence opted for an egg donation. Now, I know that my genes will not be present in my baby, and thus I am convinced that no features of the baby will resemble mine. However, I am curious to know if there's a possibility of the baby adopting some habits of mine. Will my thinking and my lifestyle during pregnancy have an affect on my baby's behaviour?

A. I find your query very touching. I am indeed confused about why you needed egg donation for PCOS. I am not sure why you were so desperate and why with treatment you could not have produced your own eggs (it is one of the commonest conditions in women and almost 20% women have PCOS). Anyway, now that you are pregnant you have the anxieties that all parents/surrogate parents share these days with all these artificial reproductive technologies. There are many ethical and medical questions which worry us. I am so glad you had the courage to share your anxieties with us.

Well, you seem disappointed that your child would not look like you but you obviously want to contribute to his/her upbringing as a parent. While it is true that your child has no genes from you, it is also true that to become the persons we finally do, we also imbibe a lot from our parents apart from genes (environmental influences). The most important thing we get from our parents (and pass on to our kids) is our value system. Nothing that you do or do not do right now, during pregnancy, will be inherited by your child (as in habits), but indeed you should keep talking to the baby in the womb as all mothers do and so should your husband. Babies get tremendous security from the mother's words and will recognize her voice (the tone and the tenor) immediately after birth (within minutes of birth). This is important in his/her feeling welcome in this world and very good for early bonding.

Another thing you can do for your child is to look after your nutrition properly, during pregnancy and breastfeeding (do not eat too much but eat healthy) so that the fetus/baby grows to his/her potential. At this, you may be better than the woman who donated an egg for you and your child may grow better because of that.

Like all couples who undergo treatment for infertility with assisted technology, I hope you too went in for counselling sessions, as depression is a commonly noted condition, especially if the first cycle is not successful. Counselling is even more important and intensive in cases like yours, when couples are planning to conceive with donor eggs, donor sperms, donor embryos, or with the help of surrogate mothers.

Your thoughts, however adverse, will not affect the baby's growth but will harm your bonding with him/her. You should stop thinking of your body as one with foreign genes. All such thoughts should have been given up once you decided to go ahead with a donor egg. Now please stop thinking about all this and enjoy your motherhood. I wish you all (you, your husband and the baby who is coming) all the best and am sure you will make a lovely family. The little one will bring tremendous joy to the family and will grow up to make his/her parents proud.

24. Why am I unhappy during my pregnancy?

Q. I am 27 years old and in the 6th month of my pregnancy. My problem is that I feel depressed and don't feel happy about my pregnancy. Although my pregnancy was planned and my husband is quite supportive, I still don't feel happy about it. I feel guilty for not being happy. I feel that no one is taking care of me and everyone is shouting at me and taunting me. I feel that no one is concerned about my well-being. Everyone tells me that I should keep happy these days but the environment around me does not seem happy at all. I keep crying all the time. My main concern is, will it affect my baby? I do shout at others but I feel they provoke me. I don't want my baby to be affected by all this. I am eating well and it's just that I am not happy. Earlier I used to be the happiest girl – I was always smiling but now I don't feel happy.

A. Sometimes pregnancy itself can precipitate depressive symptoms, due to neurohormonal changes, changes in expected roles and responsibilities, limitations in mobility and various other psychosocial and physiological changes. The stress generated by depression can affect the psychological development of the fetus, besides affecting its physical health. You should consult a psychiatrist for proper treatment and advice. Nowadays, safe treatment methods including medicines are available to curb the problem of depression during pregnancy.

Mental health should be evaluated at the first prenatal visit by the obstetrician.

Pregnancy is a major stress in life, and can unmask or exacerbate depressive tendencies. You may need a psychiatric evaluation and counselling, as women with depression are more prone to preterm labour. Depression in the postpartum period (up to 6 weeks after delivery) is also more likely in such women.

25. Will I be able to conceive with an Rh-negative factor?

Q. I am 27 years old and have a negative Rh factor – I am A negative. I conceived once but had a D&C. I did not take the rhogram injection to stop antibodies from developing in my body. I want to conceive now. Do I still have a chance of getting pregnant? Is there something I have to do? I have done a hormone test and I was told I have a high level of prolactin. Is this the cause?

A. The Rh (rhesus) factor is a protein (antigen) present on the surface of red blood cells (RBCs). As it was first discovered in the rhesus monkey, it has been so named. Individuals carrying this antigen are called Rh-positive (Rh+) while those lacking it are called Rh-negative (Rh–) blood group type. Rh incompatibility (or Rh disease) is a state in which a woman with Rh-negative blood group is exposed to Rh-positive RBCs (either by carrying an Rh-positive baby or by transfusion of Rh-positive blood) leading to the formation of antibodies (called Rh antibodies) against this protein. Once these antibodies are made in the mother, they cross the placenta during subsequent pregnancies, into the developing baby's circulation and destroy the baby's RBCs, which are Rh-positive.

When an Rh-negative woman conceives the child of an Rh-positive man, the baby may be Rh-positive. During pregnancy and delivery, red cells from the baby enter the mother's circulation. If the exposure is significant, the mother gets sensitized and begins to produce antibodies. When these antibodies cross the placenta and enter the baby's circulation, they destroy the Rh-positive cells, leading to anaemia and jaundice in the baby. Delivery is the usual time when sensitization occurs and thus, first-born babies are usually unaffected, as antibodies have not yet formed in the mother. A subsequent pregnancy with an Rh-positive baby can give rise to anaemia in the baby as these antibodies destroy the baby's RBCs. Each successive pregnancy poses a greater risk to the baby. It is postulated that even less than 1 ml of Rh-positive blood can induce antibody formation while several studies have shown that ~30% Rh-negative individuals never form antibodies despite exposure to Rh antigen.

The problem of Rh incompatibility is of clinical importance only in a pregnant woman or if blood transfusion is required. These circulating antibodies in a woman's blood are otherwise harmless. Most institutions give human anti-D immune globulin (Rh IgG) antenatally to Rh-negative pregnant women. If a woman has been already sensitized she needs to get the antibody titres estimated and be closely monitored during pregnancy. Babies born to such mothers too may require specialized neonatal care.

You should undergo blood grouping (ABO and Rh), and an antibody screen. Depending on the results of the antibody screen, mother's antibody levels and father's and/or fetal RBC antigens may need to be studied. If the fetal RBCs express the antigen against which the mother has antibodies, serial measurements of mother's antibody levels and abdominal sonograms should be done throughout the pregnancy.

It is important to know whether or not the father of the first pregnancy was/is Rh-positive. If he is Rh-negative, then there is no cause for worry.

The prolactin level is not mentioned. It is better to repeat the test to confirm it is indeed high. The test should be done early in the morning, and you should abstain from sex and exercise just prior to testing. Some women have transient or fluctuating high levels.

High prolactin can result in infertility. The cause of the high prolactin level (hyperprolactinaemia) needs to be ascertained. Common causes are hypothyroidism, stress, excessive breast stimulation, and certain drugs such as antidepressants, mood elevators, antihypertensives, metoclopramide, cimetidine, domperidone and contraceptive pills. Polycystic ovarian syndrome is associated with infertility and hyperprolactinaemia. Idiopathic hyperprolactinaemia (no cause found) can be treated with bromocriptine or cabergoline.

26. Did I have a failed pregnancy due to a negative Rh factor?

Q. I recently found that I am 7 weeks pregnant. My Rh factor is negative. I am aware of the injection I am supposed to take. But I am concerned about my past pregnancies. I have had 2 abortions and a miscarriage. Can it affect this pregnancy as well?

A. If your husband is Rh positive then there is a point of concern, especially if you have not taken the anti-D injection earlier after your two abortions and the miscarriage. I guess those previous pregnancies were from your current husband. However, if your husband is also Rh negative then there is no problem related to the Rh factor.

If your husband is Rh positive you need to undergo an indirect Coombs test (blood test), and if positive the antibody titre needs to be estimated – this test will give a good idea whether or not you have developed antibodies to the Rh-positive red blood cells, which can harm your baby if the baby you are carrying is Rh positive. These days one can also test whether or not your Rh-positive husband is homozygous or heterozygous. If he is heterozygous, there is a 50% chance your baby will be Rh negative and you need not worry. Also, some special centres are doing chorionic villus sampling (CVS) at around 10 weeks to determine whether the baby is Rh positive or Rh negative. However, the CVS procedure itself carries a 3%–5% abortion risk. So you have to weigh the pros and cons of resorting to this.

27. What should be the follicle size and endometrial thickness to become pregnant?

Q. **What should the required follicle size and endometrial thickness be before and after ovulation to become pregnant?**

A. The endometrial thickness should be at least 8 mm and follicles should be 18–25 mm in size.

28. What causes post-delivery urine retention?

Q. **I delivered my first baby earlier this month. It was a normal delivery. Due to prolonged labour of 15 hours, they gave me epidural anaesthesia, which was topped up twice after that. After the delivery, I developed urine retention. I was catheterized and discharged. My urine routine examination was 10–15 pus cells and the culture didn't reveal anything. Could it be because I was on antibiotics on and off? What could be the reason for this problem? How can this be managed? Currently I have been asked to go for clamping, urge based. What is my prognosis and how long will I take to recover?**

A. Post-delivery retention of urine is not rare. It occurs due to inability of the bladder muscles to contract and muscles sometimes take a long time to recover. Neither prolonged catheterization nor intermittent clamping is desirable in such conditions, as these manoeuvres can cause serious bladder and whole body infections (systemic sepsis). The first step in management is a thorough examination and bladder physiology evaluation with a urodynamic study. Inability of the bladder to contract, once proved, is treated with clean intermittent catheterization and some bladder contracting medications. All such cases recover, though the recovery may take long, even up to 10–12 weeks.

29. Will my breasts return to their pre-pregnancy shape?

Q. **I am 26 years old and a mother of an 8-month-old child. Will the shape of my breasts return to the pre-pregnancy state once I stop feeding my baby?**

A. The shape is not dependent on feeding but on pregnancy. There is generalized relaxation due to hormones and massive mobilization. Once you regain the tone, most of the deformity will be gone.

30. Is it safe to breastfeed during pregnancy?

Q. My baby girl is 11 months old and I am still breastfeeding at night. I am now pregnant again. Is it safe to breastfeed my baby? If yes, up to which month of pregnancy can I breastfeed my child? What are the consequences? Please give me some tips on how to stop feeding the baby. She does not like milk too much. She hardly has 1 or 2 glasses of milk in a day. Please also suggest some substitute for milk.

A. If you are pregnant, stop breastfeeding. It is a great nutritional burden for the mother to provide nutrients to the growing fetus and also to the child outside. Besides this, nipple stimulation, which occurs during suckling, can cause uterine contractions which could lead to an abortion. Please do the following:

- Slowly decrease the number of feeds over 7–10 days, first stopping night feeds, then day-time feeds.
- At night, keep the baby with the father or any other such person - she may cry for a few nights, but will slowly settle down.

Instead of milk, you can give her dahi (curd/yogurt), cheese, paneer (cottage cheese) and other milk products.

31. Is it normal for breast milk to leak before delivery?

Q. I am 7-and-a-half months pregnant and have noticed that my breasts are leaking milk, about 1–2 drops since the 5th month. But for past 3–4 days it is increasingly leaking more, even wetting my dress. Is this normal or am I producing milk earlier? Will it continue till my delivery or will I stop producing milk because my breast is not being suckled? Kindly advise.

A. It is not unusual to have some milk being produced before the baby is born. If the amount is large and increasing, please mention it to your doctor at your next antenatal visit.

Pregnant women should not have breast stimulation by their spouses. This can lead to preterm labour, and 'milk leaking'.

32. What is the reason for heavy and irregular periods after delivery?

Q. I am a 24-year-old female with a 2-year-old son. I had a caesarean

delivery and my appendix was also removed 4 years back. I have a problem of delayed and painful period from the beginning. After my delivery I got my first period after one year (around a year ago). Initially, my periods were almost regular. However, since the last couple of months they have again become irregular and the last time they came after the doctor prescribed some tablets. This time too it is delayed by three weeks. Also, they are painful. Presently, I have pain in the lower abdomen quite often. I have seen a doctor and she has prescribed several tests including ultrasound of the lower abdomen and pelvis. The reports are as follows: Ultrasound (lower abdomen and pelvis) – Uterus measures 66x34 mm, Endometrial thickness of 7.3 mm, Left ovary normal, Right adenexa reveals 23x31 mm tubo-ovarian (T.O.) mass. No free fluid in pelvis, Urinary bladder shows no filling defect, No wall thickening or echogenic debris seen. So the opinion is: a small right adenexal T.O. mass. Is it a tumour which needs surgery? How can it be treated? Will it ever get dissolved? The other blood tests done were for thyroid which was normal, Mantoux test was negative, ESR – 38 (normal is 0–20), S. prolactin – 5.2 (normal is 8.4–20.2). Kindly advise me whether it is a very serious problem and how it can be treated?

A. You seem to have many complaints which may or may not be related. Heavy periods and irregular periods generally have different reasons. If you have this problem after delivery at your age, heavy periods are more likely to be due to infection of the lining of the uterus called endometritis and a course of antibiotics is all you may need. Endometritis is the commonest complication of a caesarean section and as many as 70% of women who have a caesarean section have some infection in the lining of the uterus. I suggest you take a course of broad-spectrum antibiotics if your gynaecologist/obstetrician agrees with the possibility of infection. These infections can be persistent and can be very nagging and a repeat course of antibiotics may be required a few months later.

You may also have pelvic infection of some sort and the most classical sign of this is painful sex. I wonder if you have it. If you do, it is almost certainly due to a pelvic infection.

The ultrasound report you have described is not very precise. By definition, to call a mass an adenexal mass, it should be at least 5 cm thick and generally anything smaller than 3 cm (30 mm) is not due to a disease. So I do not know what to make out of it. Water-filled cysts of around 30 mm are common and occur all the time in a woman's life and they disappear on their own. They are of no consequence and do not need an ultrasound to make a diagnosis.

The cause of delayed periods will have to be looked into. By the way, are you still breastfeeding the child (which may cause irregular periods and heavy ones)? Long cycles are rarely due to a serious disease and please get investigated only if it persists more than six months or so. Chronic ill health and stress can cause delayed periods. And if your periods are delayed they would definitely be a little heavy. For example, if you have periods after 2 months they would be one-and-a-half times heavier (if not twice) than if your periods come monthly because the lining of the uterus accumulates inside and you will have a heavier prolonged period.

Since your thyroid is normal and there is no evidence of any other cause on ultrasound like polycystic ovarian syndrome (PCOS) you should not worry too much about delayed cycles at this point. (*See also* page 18)

33. Why have I not been successful in conceiving by IVF, using the ICSI technique?

Q. I have been trying to conceive by IVF using the ICSI technique. My partner has had a vasectomy and the sperm was taken directly from the testis. I have had three full cycles with good fertilization rates but no pregnancy occurred. I fear that I have an implantation problem although my uterus lining has always been above the required thickness. Does my partner's sperm have to be of good quality? Could this be the reason that I have not conceived yet? I have a history of endometriosis diagnosed by a laparoscopy four years ago, when I had a chocolate cyst removed. I have been diagnosed with another chocolate cyst, which I will get removed in some time.

A. The initial tests done on an infertile couple are based on the findings from the history and physical examination. These include testing for: ovulatory function; male factors; tubal disease; cervical disease, uterine disease and excluding endocrinal (hormonal) abnormalities/problems.

Assisted reproductive techniques include:

1. **Gamete intra-fallopian transfer (GIFT)**, designed for women with unexplained infertility. During this procedure, the patient undergoes a controlled ovarian hyperstimulation, the oocytes are retrieved transvaginally under ultrasound guidance, and 3–4 oocytes are placed via laparoscopy into one of the fallopian tubes along with sperms.

2. **Zygote intra-fallopian transfer (ZIFT)** is used for couples with a significant male cause for infertility. The oocytes are retrieved similar to GIFT, but they are allowed to fertilize *in vitro* in the laboratory. At the 2-pronuclear stage (usually 24 hours later), 3–4 embryos are transferred via laparoscopy into one of the fallopian tubes. If the embryos are allowed to develop to greater than a 2-cell stage, the procedure is termed tubal embryo transfer (TET). The only advantage of a ZIFT or TET versus the more traditional IVF is that women, who are thought to have compromised embryo quality due to embryo culture *in vitro*, now have the benefit of developing these zygotes or embryos in their own 'natural incubators'. This is thought to enhance subsequent development, with improved pregnancy rates.
3. **Intracytoplasmic sperm injection (ICSI)** is the treatment of choice for couples in whom the male partner has azoospermia or severe oligospermia. ICSI is also indicated for men with significant anti-sperm antibodies, low sperm motility, or significantly abnormal sperm morphology or when poor fertilization occurs with regular insemination techniques in the laboratory. Sperm can be obtained from the ejaculate or directly from the epididymis.

Your treating physician is best placed to advise if you can also go for another technique.

In your case, endometriosis could be contributing to implantation failure. Poor sperm quality could be a factor in failure of ICSI.

34. How does one get rid of stretch marks after pregnancy?

Q. Nine weeks ago, we had our first children – twins. My wife, who is of small build, has swollen up a lot. In addition, she has huge stretch marks. She was given a lot of iron and other vitamins as necessary during pregnancy. She also has a lot of pigmentation for which she has been advised to take B-complex capsules. How does she get rid of the stretch marks? Will she lose the pigmentation on her skin or will it be that way forever? When is the best time to start exercising again?

A. In many women the midline of the abdominal skin becomes markedly pigmented (linea nigra). Sometimes brown patches of varying sizes appear on the face and neck (mask of pregnancy), on the breasts and genital skin. These usually disappear or regress considerably after delivery. Oral contraceptive pills and sunlight aggravate these pigmented patches. Sunscreen lotions should be used on the face and neck. If the pigmentation is disfiguring, a dermatologist should be consulted.

For stretch marks, apply a vitamin E-containing cream such as Aloe vera cream.

Light exercises can be started 24 hours after a normal vaginal delivery in a healthy woman. Other exercises can be started after 2–3 weeks after normal vaginal delivery (NVD) and after 4 weeks of a CS. The exact timing would depend upon the general condition of the mother at that time. It is important to be examined by the gynaecologist/obstetrician before starting any formal exercises. It is good to consult a physiotherapist and do the exercises under his/her guidance.

35. Is it necessary to remove the clothes before a caesarean?

Q. My friend had a delivery through caesarean section. She had a very horrifying experience. She was fully stripped before her delivery, although she was given anaesthesia only on the lower part of the body. There were a lot of male helpers in the operating room. Is it necessary to strip the patient before surgery? Can the presence of male helpers be avoided? I am carrying a baby myself and don't want to get into this situation.

A. Caesarean section is a major operation. Even though the anaesthesia is given to the lower half, the abdomen is prepped with an antiseptic solution till the rib cage, for which the clothes have to be removed. However, if done sensitively, it can avoid undue embarrassment. Usually, a female attendant does this, although it may be impossible to ask all male medical and paramedical personnel to leave the operation theatre. In your case, you may discuss these concerns with your obstetrician beforehand, so that your embarrassment can be minimized.

36. Can dental treatment be done during pregnancy?

Q. My wife is 7 months pregnant. She has dental problems and needs teeth realignment, extraction for 2 or 3 and a root canal. We visited an orthodontist who says treatment will not have any impact on the pregnancy. Currently, he will extract a few teeth and fix the clip for 6–12 months. But our obstetrician

recommends no local anaesthesia and antibiotics at this stage. What is suggested in this situation?

A. I think you can wait for 4 more months and then go ahead for the treatment. Though dental treatment is not contraindicated during pregnancy, it is better not to create situations of pain or stress during this time.

37. Can a tooth be extracted during pregnancy?

Q. My wife is suffering from severe toothache. This is because of the growth of a wisdom tooth, which is covered by the gum. Since she is pregnant, the doctor has advised her not to remove the tooth. If at all they have to extract the tooth, they have to cut the gum, which is not advisable. This happened once during her 3rd month of pregnancy. Now she is in her 7th month of pregnancy. This pain usually comes at night. She feels better after taking the medicine prescribed by the doctor. But the pain starts again after some time. Can the tooth be removed now?

A. The tooth can usually be safely extracted in the second trimester of pregnancy. The final decision will be that of the treating gynaecologist/ obstetrician and the treating dental surgeon. The gum can be safely cauterized at this point of time.

38. What are the causes of low TSH during pregnancy?

Q. During a blood test last week for confirming pregnancy, the report said that my wife's TSH level is 0.02 which is very much lower than the normal level of 0.24. Her other readings for Free T4 and Total T4 are normal and within the ranges. What are the reasons for this and what precautions does she need?

A. This condition is known as subclinical hyperthyroidism and can occur in early pregnancy in women having excessive vomiting due to human chorionic gonadotrophin (hCG) hormone from the placenta. Observation is all right if your wife is pregnant but repeat tests should be done after 4–6 weeks. Hyperthyroidism is a condition in which there is excessive thyroid hormone production in the body.

39. Can a pregnant woman take alcohol?

Q. Can a pregnant woman drink wine? If yes, what should be the quantity and frequency?

A. It is advisable not to have any kind of alcohol during pregnancy. So try not to have any kind of alcohol. In case you have to take it, then only 2–3 times during the 9 months and that too only 1–2 pegs. (*See also* page 13)

40. Why do I have pain in the lower back and buttocks after pregnancy?

Q. I am a 30-year-old mother of two children. During my second pregnancy, I developed stiffness and pain in my lower back and hips. This continued after delivery as well. Now my child is 9 months old. The doctor diagnosed it as a type of arthritis, which develops during pregnancy and is completely curable. I am on a painkiller now, and my pain still continues. Is this type of arthritis really curable? Will I have to bear the pain and further complications in future? Are there any specific exercises which will improve my condition?

A. Spinal problems can generally be categorized into two types.

1. The common form of strain–sprain–posture related ordinary back pain. Ninety per cent of the low back pain belongs to this category. It is nothing serious. Simple posture correction and exercises for strengthening the muscles of the back (to be learnt from an occupational therapist or physiotherapist) and reassurance (that it is not life-threatening or serious) is all that is needed. Occasionally paracetamol (the safest and simplest painkiller) along with some muscle relaxant (for example, amytriptyline 10 mg, 2 hours before going to bed) is all that is needed.

2. The serious type of spinal arthritis – inflammatory or immunological in nature – requires correct diagnosis and the latest treatment with modern medicines. For this you would have to take the advice of a rheumatologist (physician specializing in joint diseases). He/she would assess you for inflammatory spinal disease (called spondyloarthritis or ankylosing spondylitis) and then treat you accordingly.

Diet and nutrition

41. How much weight should be gained during pregnancy?

Q. I am a 29-year-old married woman and am very lean and underweight for my height. I am expecting a baby in the next couple of months. What are the chances of the baby being underweight, and will it be healthy?

A. You need to take vitamins and eat a healthy nutritious diet. You need to gain between 20 and 30 pounds during pregnancy. If your weight gain is adequate, then your pre-pregnancy weight is not as important, provided it is above 45 kg. However, a woman with a pre-pregnancy weight of less than 45 kg is considered at risk for complications during pregnancy for herself and her baby.

The recommended total weight gain for women carrying a single baby is as follows:

Pre-pregnancy BMI	Recommended total gain (pound)	Recommended total gain (kilogram)
Low (BMI <19.8)	28–40	12.5–18
Normal (BMI 19.8–25)	25–35	11.5–16
High (BMI >26–29)	15–25	7–11.5
Obese (BMI >29)	<15	<7

Source: IFIC Foundation, 2003

The range for women with twins is 35–45 lb (16–20 kg).
The increase for women with triplets is 50 lb (23 kg).

$$\text{BMI} = \text{body mass index} = \frac{\text{weight (in kg)}}{\text{height } (\text{m}^2)} \times 100$$

The target weight gain in women with a normal BMI is 0.4 kg per week during the second and third trimesters (especially after 20 weeks); in women with low BMI the target weight gain is 0.5 kg per week after 20 weeks; and the target weight gain in those with a high BMI is 0.3 kg per week in the second and third trimesters.

42. Why is there weight loss in pregnancy?

Q. My wife has completed 4 months of pregnancy. In her recent health check-up visit, she found that she has lost around 3 kg since her last check-up two months back. Even though she has completed 4 months she is still throwing up and despite having Doxinate according to the doctor's prescription, there is no improvement. This is her second pregnancy. In her first pregnancy, she did not have nausea.

A. Losing 3 kg in the first half of the pregnancy is not alarming. Most women lose 1–3 kg between the 2nd and the 5th months. There are various reasons for it but for now it may suffice to say that it is normal and you should not worry about it. The nausea should have settled by now or maybe it will in the next few weeks.

The causes of nausea during pregnancy are not fully understood and therefore it cannot be cured. The best you can do is to make your wife as comfortable as possible. There are a few things which you should keep in mind.

- The nausea of pregnancy is a trigger and will only get worse once it starts in the morning.
- The triggers of nausea are many and vary from person to person. You will have to identify the objects, smells and taste, even the thoughts, which cause nausea in your wife. It could be something you eat or drink or even a perfume. It is not necessarily an allergy, i.e. you may suddenly start hating something that you have loved all your life – such as a perfume or a particular food.
- The commonest nausea-inducing agent in the early morning is toothpaste. So while your wife has to brush her teeth last thing in the night, she doesn't necessarily have to do it first thing in the morning (something we all do but may not be essential). She can rinse her mouth with plain water or with the toothbrush without paste.

- An empty stomach, especially in the morning, triggers nausea. She must take a small bite as soon as she gets up. Let her take a small biscuit in bed and maybe a cup of tea or coffee.
- Cooking smells are another potent cause of nausea, so are petrol fumes and extremes of temperature. Long journeys would also be uncomfortable.

Basically, you have to identify the agents that trigger nausea in your wife and avoid that agent, even if you have to be rude like asking someone not to smoke in her presence.

The drugs given (such as Doxinate) can be helpful but do not fully cure nausea. If it has not helped so far it is unlikely that it will help now. (I hope your wife is taking the drug properly and at the right time. Please check with your doctor whether she is taking the right dose.)

It is interesting that you say that the nausea was not there in the last pregnancy. This can happen. The second pregnancy is more symptomatic, meaning that it causes more symptoms (such as backache, nausea, weakness) though it has fewer complications (e.g. hypertension and low birth weight) than the first pregnancy. This is contrary to the normal perception. Again, there are a lot of theories about this. As I said, we do not know why nausea occurs so we cannot really explain why it is more in the second pregnancy, but we assume it is because of some kind of an allergic response to the father's proteins (half of the baby's proteins come from the father's genes). For all allergies, prior exposure to the protein is required. This partly explains why there are more symptoms in the second pregnancy as compared with the first.

While she has nausea she has to be careful about her eating habits during this part of the pregnancy. Do not worry too much about nutrition at this stage of the pregnancy. In other words, there are no good or bad foods of pregnancy. There should be no force-feeding and no restrictions. Food that does not bring on nausea is good food for your wife and vice versa. However nutritious a food may be, e.g. milk or green vegetables, if it causes nausea in your wife, please do not ask her to take it. As long as the food is not infected (bought from outside) it is all right, however 'un-nutritious' it may be. She does not have to eat too much. Whatever she is able to eat is good enough. If she forces herself to eat beyond this, it will only cause vomiting. If she cannot eat anything at all even then it is all right as long as she has plenty of fluids to avoid dehydration.

Food tips:

1. Take a meal every hour or two throughout the day.
2. Breakfast should be taken an hour or more after getting up and take an early pre-lunch snack at around 11 a.m.
3. Lunch should be followed by a late afternoon snack and evening tea followed by an early dinner.
4. All meals of the day should be small.
5. Do not eat too much and do not starve.

Frequent, small meals is the rule. Eating too much at one time will cause vomiting and remaining hungry would lead to nausea. I hope this adequately answers your doubts.

43. Why is my weight decreasing during pregnancy?

Q. I am 14 weeks and 2 days pregnant. My problem is that my weight seems to be decreasing. I started with 64 kg, and by the 11th week it was 63 kg. It went up to 63.5 kg in the 13th week, but now it is 61 kg. At present, I am 3 kg less than that at the start of my pregnancy. I wanted to check if this indicates any serious problem. My blood results have not come yet, but the scan at the 12th week showed that the baby is of the right size. Could you please advise?

A. Some weight loss is common in the initial weeks, especially if you have experienced a fair amount of morning sickness. Since the baby appears to be growing appropriately, I would not be overly concerned. This said, I would still encourage you to eat a healthy, well-balanced diet with extra calories for the baby. If your weight does not start going up in the next few weeks, you should consult a nutritionist.

44. How can one gain weight during pregnancy?

Q. I am 6-and-a-half months pregnant (second pregnancy). For the past 2-and-a-half months my weight is not increasing. Initially, before conceiving, my weight was 62 kg. After 3 months of pregnancy, my weight came down to 61.5 kg. Now, after 6 months of pregnancy, my weight is 65 kg. So, from the date of conceiving till now, my weight has increased by 3 kg only. My height is 5.3 inches. I got an ultrasound scan done during the 21st week. The report indicated a fetus of 23 weeks. There is no other problem as such. Although

the baby is large for date as per the scanning report, my caregiver is a little worried about my constant weight. She has suggested some tonics, tablets and proteins and I am taking them regularly. Also, I would like to inform you that I am a working woman and I don't find time to eat sufficiently. As I am completing 7 months, is it necessary for me to take maternity leave from now itself, so that I can eat properly and take rest, in order to increase my weight? Could you kindly let me know whether this constant weight affects my baby's growth?

A. Your baby's growth seems to be all right. It is possible that you are not gaining weight because you are not taking a proper diet. You should eat every 2–3 hours. Take a good, nutritious diet that includes green vegetables, fruits and milk products. Supplement the diet with vitamins, proteins, calcium and iron. Plenty of working women keep working till just before delivery. You may continue to do that. But do take proper rest – at least 8–10 hours of sleep every day.

45. What precautions do I need to take for my rapid weight gain during pregnancy?

Q. I am 26 years old and I weighed 65 kg before pregnancy. My weight was 84 kg in the beginning of the 9th month. The weight gain was normal at 75 kg up to the 7th month. After that it remained at 80 kg in the 8th month. The amniotic fluid was low, i.e. oligohydramnios in the 8th month. After taking dextrose intravenously 3 times on alternate days, the weight increased by 4 kg. I am taking vitamin and iron tablets regularly as suggested by the doctor as I seem to have polycystic ovarian syndrome (PCOS). I have a hormonal problem. Is the weight gain normal in my case? I have been advised to undergo an ultrasound scan (the third time in 20 days). I had swelling on the legs and arms in the 8th month but it reduced later. My blood pressure is normal at around 110–120/70–80 mmHg. The baby is in the head-down position now and it changed from a breech position in the 34th week. What precautions do I need to take for my weight and in general?

A. It appears that you have gained significant weight in this pregnancy. I would recommend that you follow your doctor's advice on ultrasounds to monitor the oligohydramnios and your blood pressure.

In general, eating many fruits, vegetables, proteins and avoiding fried foods and sweets will keep your weight under control. Also avoid excess salt. It makes you retain fluid. Please keep up with monitoring of your blood pressure. Any significant rise in the blood pressure in conjunction with your rapid weight gain may point towards pre-eclampsia. Unless your gynaecologist/obstetrician recommends rest, I will suggest walking for some time to keep the weight down; it may also help to have an easier delivery. Make sure you drink plenty of fluids and milk to maintain hydration.

46. Can refrigerated foods be taken during pregnancy?

Q. If a pregnant woman takes refrigerated foods regularly, what effect will it have on the baby?

A. Refrigerated foods *per se* are unlikely to cause any adverse effect on the baby. A balanced diet with adequate nutrients is the key issue. As long as fresh fruits and vegetables along with dairy products and grains are being consumed (refrigerated or not), there should be no problem. Spoilt and stale food should be strictly avoided. Whatever supplements are prescribed by your doctor must be consumed regularly.

47. Is it harmful to drink tea during pregnancy?

Q. I want to know if tea is harmful during pregnancy, especially in the first trimester.

A. It is suggested to restrict the caffeine intake from tea and coffee during pregnancy and lactation. You can have 2 cups of tea per day during pregnancy.

48. How much calcium does a pregnant woman require?

Q. I am 32 weeks pregnant and I want to know whether taking too much calcium is harmful in any way. I take calcium tablets of 500 mg per day and 2 glasses of orange juice, 2 glasses of milk, and 1 cup of yogurt every day.

A. An inadequate amount of calcium intake is associated with low birth-weight babies, pre-eclampsia and bone pains in the mother.

The calcium requirement of a pregnant woman is 1 g/day (1000 mg/day). The total of all the sources which you have mentioned is a little more than this figure (your calcium intake is approximately 1200 mg/day). Calcium overload can cause potential health hazards only if its consumption is as high as 2500 mg/day. Calcium is an important nutrient for the healthy growth of your baby's bones; hence meeting its requirement is very important. You can carry on with your dietary regimen without any worry.

49. Can I eat or drink sugar-free products during pregnancy?

Q. I am 21 years old. Can I drink or eat sugar-free foods during pregnancy?

A. There are two categories of sweeteners: nutritive (contain calories) and non-nutritive (without calories). Nutritive sweeteners (such as table sugar, honey, corn sugar, etc.) contain what is called 'empty' calories. These additives contribute calories to the diet, but they also contain a few vitamins or minerals. However, women with carbohydrate intolerance such as gestational diabetes, diabetes mellitus or insulin resistance need to limit their use of nutritive sweeteners. In foods labelled as 'sugar-free', we find sugar alcohols, which are also nutritive sweeteners. Technically, sugar alcohols are not sugars, but they do have calories, which can be converted into fat. Examples of sugar alcohols include: sorbitol, xylitol, isomalt, mannitol and hydrogenated starch.

Non-nutritive sweeteners are added in very small amounts to foods for a significant sweetening effect and have been approved for use in diabetic or reduced calorie foods and beverages.

The following are non-nutritive sweeteners that are considered safe during pregnancy:

Acesulfame potassium (Sunett): This sweetener is added to baked goods, frozen desserts, sugar-free gelatines, puddings and beverages. This is considered safe to use in moderation during pregnancy by the US Food and Drug Administration (FDA).

Aspartame (Equal or NutraSweet): Aspartame is not effective at high temperatures or for long periods in liquid form. It is often found as an additive in soft drinks, gelatine, desserts, pudding mixes, breakfast cereals, beverages, chewing gum, dairy products, and other foods and drugs. According to the FDA, aspartame is safe for use during pregnancy and lactation. It is, however, recommended to limit consumption to a moderate level.

Aspartame should not be used by anyone with phenylketonuria (PKU) (a rare metabolic disorder), rare liver disease, or by pregnant women who have high levels of phenylalanine in their blood. Phenylalanine is a component of aspartame, and it may not metabolize correctly in anyone who has these conditions.

Sucralose (Splenda, SugarFree): This is a non-caloric sweetener that is made from sugar. Sucralose has been approved for use in baked goods, baking mixes, non-alcoholic beverages, chewing gum, coffee and tea products, confections and frostings, fats and oils, frozen dairy desserts and mixes, fruit juices, sugar substitutes, sweet sauces, toppings and syrups. It can also be used as a 'table-top sweetener'. Sucralose has no effect on blood sugar, offers no calories, and is deemed safe during pregnancy and lactation. According to the FDA, sucralose is safe for everyone to consume, including pregnant women.

Avoid the use of the following:

Cyclamate: Cyclamate is not considered safe for anyone including pregnant women.

Saccharine (Sweet N Low): Although it is not used as much today as in the past, it still appears in many foods, beverages and other substances. Saccharine crosses the placenta and may be a risk for pregnant women. High saccharine exposure *in utero* and throughout life have been linked to increased risk of bladder cancer.

Stevia: This sweetener is derived from a shrub. It can add sweetness to foods, but has been banned by the FDA as a sweetener.

If you use artificial sweeteners and are pregnant, it is always best to have a talk with your doctor about which sweetener you should use and how much you should consume. Preferably avoid all forms of artificial food during pregnancy.

50. What is the quantity of vitamin A and D required by a pregnant woman?

Q. Is it true that cod liver oil tablets are a good source of omega-3 fatty acids and are good for general health? I have bought the Walgreens brand of tablets and each tablet has 1250 IU of vitamin A (25% daily value) and 135 IU of vitamin D (34% daily value). I have a cup of milk every day. Will these tablets cause an overdose of vitamins A and D? How much exposure to sunlight provides enough vitamin D for the day? Will I have to buy another pack of cod liver oil tablets without vitamin supplements? Gynaecologists recommend folic acid for women planning to conceive. Is it safe to have both these tablets?

A. There is a widespread misconception that vitamin supplements are always helpful and never harmful. Nothing could be further from the truth. Unfortunately, companies manufacturing vitamin supplements, because of their commercial interest in selling their products, are as much at fault as the people who consume them.

Normal healthy people adequately meet the daily requirements of vitamin A and D from normal food and sunlight. There is absolutely no need for vitamin supplements. Intake of high doses of vitamin A leads to side-effects including abnormalities in the fetus. High intake of vitamin D leads to high calcium levels in the blood, which in turn causes congenital defects in babies.

Vitamin D synthesis occurs in the body by normal exposure to sunlight in our day-to-day life. There is absolutely no need to expose oneself to sunlight especially for this purpose.

Women planning pregnancy should take iron and folic acid (e.g. Fecontin-F Continus), 1 tablet daily till labour.

The recommended daily allowance (RDA) of vitamin A is:

- For non-pregnant women: 600 mcg RE
- For pregnant women: 600 mcg RE
- For lactating women: 950 mcg RE

(1 RE [Retinol equivalent] = 6 μg of beta carotene; 1 μg of retinol; =3.33 IU)

A normal, healthy woman takes sufficient amounts of vitamin A in the regular diet in the form of butter, green and yellow vegetables, and yellow fruits. Lack of vitamin A can lead to blindness, decreased brain development in the baby and a defective immune system. High intake through supplements (>10,000 units per day) can cause malformations in the baby.

The RDA of vitamin D is:

- For non-pregnant women: 5 mcg
- For pregnant women: 10 mcg
- For lactating women: 10 mcg

Normally, a person has sufficient stores of vitamin D as it is mainly synthesized in the skin by exposure to sunlight. It is also present in fortified milk and margarine, fish liver and oil. It is toxic to the fetus in excessive amounts. On the other hand, infants born to mothers with vitamin D deficiency have delayed bone ossification and defective enamel formation (of the teeth).

Omega-3 fatty acid is the predominant structural fatty acid of the brain and retina (eye). The International Society for the Study of Fats and Lipids (ISSFAL) recommends an intake of 220 mg per day of omega-3 fatty acid for adults and 300 mg per day for pregnant and lactating women. Fish and fish oil, some seeds and oils, green leafy vegetables, walnuts and soyabeans are rich in omega-3 fatty acids. Supplementation of the maternal diet with omega-3 fatty acids during the periconceptional period, pregnancy and lactation is beneficial for the development of the brain and visual acuity of the baby.

The RDA of folic acid is:

- For non-pregnant women: 180 mcg
- For pregnant women: 400 mcg
- For lactating women: 280 mcg

Liver, leafy vegetables and yeast are rich in folic acid. Deficiency of folic acid can lead to anaemia. Folic acid supplementation of 400 mcg per day prior to conception helps in reducing neural tube defects in the baby.

51. Is the consumption of silver leaf on sweets harmful during pregnancy?

Q. I am in my 21st week of pregnancy. I have been consuming 2–3 *kaju* rolls everyday. Is the silver leaf (*chandi warak*), which is on the *kaju* roll/*burfi* safe during pregnancy? Is it harmful for fetal development?

A. There is no direct link found between silver leaf intake in the quantity you mention and harmful effects during pregnancy. However, in your physiological condition, I would prefer that you do not take this and also not worry. Consult your doctor if you note any gastrointestinal symptoms.

52. How can I improve my iron and calcium levels through diet?

Q. I am 4 months pregnant and my doctor has prescribed a high dosage of

iron and calcium tablets. My haemoglobin is 13.3. I have been taking wheat, *ragi* and rice daily with three types of fruits: apple, banana and pomegranate. I also take a lot of green leafy vegetables, pulses and dry fruits such as almonds, apricot and dates. I hate to take tablets. How can I substitute these tablets through natural sources of iron and calcium?

A. When the level of haemoglobin (Hb) is not adequate, according to the age and sex of an individual, he or she is said to be suffering from anaemia. It is diagnosed in pregnant women when the haemoglobin level is less than 11.5 g/dl. Anaemia is twice as common in women than in men, especially during the childbearing years, due to menstrual blood loss and pregnancy. The most common cause of anaemia in pregnancy is deficiency of iron (~85% cases) and folic acid. Even if a woman is not anaemic at the time of pregnancy, she may still develop anaemia as the pregnancy progresses due to increased demand by the developing baby. There are certain risk factors for the development of anaemia in pregnant women and these include: poor nutrition, inadequate gap between pregnancies, persistent nausea or vomiting in early pregnancy and twin pregnancy.

The loss of iron (elemental) with each normal menstrual period is around 12–15 mg. A normal diet must include 1.5–2 mg/day of elemental iron to compensate for menstrual losses alone. In pregnancy, 500 mg of additional iron is needed by the mother (to expand her red cell mass) while another 500 mg is needed for the baby and placental tissues. Thus, on an average, an additional 3 mg/day of elemental iron must be absorbed from dietary sources. Iron is obtained from foods in our diet but only 1 mg of iron is absorbed for every 10 to 20 mg of iron ingested (i.e. the amount of iron absorbed by the body is only 10% of the total amount consumed), thus 30 mg/day needs to be consumed to meet the requirement.

Absorption of iron from food is influenced by multiple factors. One important factor is the form of the iron. Iron in foods comes in two forms haem-iron (meat, poultry, fish) and non-haem or inorganic iron (vegetable source). Haem-iron is highly available for absorption in contrast to non-haem iron. Vegetarians need more iron in their diet than non-vegetarians because the iron from plant foods is not as well absorbed as it is from animal foods. Vegetarians should choose several iron-rich plant foods daily. Grains, beans and lentils, vegetables (green-leafy ones, tomato, potato, green and red chillies, etc.), fruits, nuts and seeds are rich sources of non-haem iron. Apples, bananas, brinjals (aubergine or egg plant), and jaggery are rich sources of iron. Ascorbic acid (vitamin C) and foods rich in this vitamin (citrus fruits) enhance the absorption of iron.

The absorption of non-haem iron can be improved when a source of haem-iron (meat, fish and poultry) or iron absorption-enhancing foods (fruits or fruit juices) is consumed in the same meal. On the other hand, coffee, tea and calcium impair iron absorption if consumed along with a meal, as do inhibitors such as bran, vegetable fibre and phosphates. You will need to restrict your consumption of milk so that you have an adequate appetite for iron-containing foods as milk does not contain any iron.

It is for these reasons that all pregnant women are given iron and folic acid supplementation.

Milk, cheese, curd, ice cream, egg yolk, fish, whole grains, cereals (especially *ragi*), and green leafy vegetables (spinach and amaranth) are important sources of calcium. Milk and milk products are the best sources of dietary calcium. A litre of cow's milk contains about 1200 mg of calcium. About 20%–30% of calcium is absorbed from the total calcium in our diet. Absorption of calcium is enhanced by vitamin D, and decreased by the presence of phytates (in cereals), oxalates (in green leafy vegetables) and fatty acids in the diet. Therefore, all pregnant women require calcium supplements.

The RDA (recommended dietary allowance) for Indian women is as follows:

	Iron	Calcium
Non-pregnant	30 mg/day	400 mg/day
Pregnant	38 mg/day	1000 mg/day
Lactating	30 mg/day	1000 mg/day

53. Which foods should be avoided during pregnancy?

Q. I am 10 weeks pregnant. I would like to know which fruits and vegetables I should avoid.

A. You must take a well-balanced diet, which meets your requirements, as well as that of the growing fetus. There are no foods as such that you need to avoid but it depends on each individual's tolerance. Some women are unable to tolerate milk and milk products while others may not be able to tolerate acidic foods and fruits. You can find out for yourself which foods cause acidity and nausea in your case, and try to avoid them for some time. However, do not avoid any such food totally, rather try them again after a few days and include them if tolerated well. Do not force feed yourself and plan out a diet, depending on your likes and dislikes to make it more appealing, after 20 weeks of pregnancy.

54. Can dieting affect pregnancy?

Q. My problem is that I get tired often. I keep yawning even when I am not tired. I would like to know the reason for this. I am overweight for my height and would like to diet. I am trying to conceive. But I read that dieting just before you conceive may have an adverse effect on the child. Is this true? I have developed a paunch because of my weight (my tummy was on the bigger side even when I was slim) and I also feel a slight trace of constant pain in my lower abdomen. I do not know whether all these symptoms are interconnected. Please comment about my symptoms and recommend whether I need to contact any specialist.

A. Tiredness is a common complaint, with numerous possible causes. However, a more common problem is the vicious circle caused by the tired person failing to exercise sufficiently: this leads to muscles becoming deconditioned, and then effort becomes more demanding, thus increasing the feeling of tiredness. The initial step would be to increase exercise (e.g. walk fast for half an hour a day) and go on a stricter diet that limits carbohydrate intake, but favours an increased fibre intake. This could also help the bowels and reduce abdominal discomfort. Dieting will not have an adverse effect on pregnancy, especially if added vitamins – including folic acid – are taken regularly.

55. Is curd a good substitute for milk during pregnancy? Does papaya cause miscarriages?

Q. I am currently in my 4th month of pregnancy. I take a full diet along with fruits and curd. I cannot digest milk and after taking milk I cannot have any other food, and I get nauseous. But I take curd regularly – twice a day. Do you think taking curd in place of milk is sufficient as its substitute? Among fruits, I love papaya a lot. But I have gone through some foreign and Indian websites. It has been suggested not to take papaya in pregnancy as it leads to abortion. Do you think this is correct? I already had one miscarriage last year.

A. You do not need milk, as milk is probably not good for you; milk is also not essential at this stage of pregnancy (or at any other stage). Milk is one good source of calcium but curd or cheese are good substitutes. Any food that makes you sick should be avoided. If milk makes you sick, avoid it; milk in the form of curd is not only as good but probably better as it is easier to digest.

You say you are taking a full diet – I hope this means you are taking a healthy balanced diet without too many raw calories in the form of fats and sugars. What you need is a balanced diet including proteins, minerals and vitamins and not high calorie foods which have a reputation of being pregnancy foods. There are no good or bad foods of pregnancy. Eat what you like and as much as you like. Just be careful about the quality of food.

Whatever you have eaten all your life is normal diet for you. Needless to say, you should take a balanced diet, but try not to be too stressed about it (and tell concerned people around you and in your family not to worry too much about it).

There should be no force-feeding and no restrictions. All food which does not bring on nausea is good food for you. However nutritious a food may be, such as milk or green vegetables, if it causes nausea, please do not take it. You do not have to eat too much. Whatever you are able to eat is good enough. If you force yourself to eat more than you can, it will only cause vomiting. It is also all right even if you cannot eat anything at all as long as you have plenty of fluids to prevent dehydration.

It is a myth that papaya causes abortion. I do not know the origin of this myth but it seems to be universal. Perhaps its capacity to cause motion gives an impression that it will carry the fetus down somehow. However, there is no scientific evidence in favour of this myth, and taken in moderation it causes no harm and may actually be good in countering constipation, if you have it.

56. Can lemon juice, coconut milk and guava affect my pregnancy?

Q. I am 13 weeks pregnant. Before pregnancy I used to take lemon juice twice a day with sugar, and after pregnancy I now take lemon juice with salt, not very regularly but immediately after vomiting. I have been told that pregnant women should not drink lemon juice. Is this correct? As I have been taking it for nearly 13 weeks, is this going to affect my baby or me? Now I drink the water of a tender coconut twice a day – once in the morning as

soon as I wake up and once in the evening. Can I continue with that? I also eat more guavas as compared with other fruits, is that all right? One of our relatives who took a lot of lemon juice and guavas got white patches all over her body after her delivery. Could that be due to lemon and/or guavas? Please advise on the foods that I can have.

A. Fruits are good at all times. Fruits such as guava and lemon juice do not have anything to do with white patches. Tender coconut juice is also good. However, too much of anything may cause problems. You must have a balanced diet. By now your vomiting would have stopped. A diet rich in fibre is good. The fruits and juices in the quantities you have mentioned will not harm your baby.

57. Will eating raw garlic affect my pregnancy?

Q. I am 28 years old, weight 65 kg and am planning a pregnancy. I have high blood pressure (BP). Can I have raw garlic every day in the morning, during pregnancy? Will it affect my pregnancy?

A. Garlic does not create any problem during pregnancy but it is not the right and the only way to reduce blood pressure. In case you are still planning a pregnancy, you first need to reduce your weight in a healthy way so as to assist your pregnancy. Along with weight loss you should reduce salt intake, and do some exercises and yoga to reduce your blood pressure.

58. Is it safe to consume ginger *ladoos* during pregnancy?

Q. During which month of pregnancy is it safe to consume ginger *ladoos* and what is the suggested number a pregnant woman can consume in a day?

A. Ginger is generally used for morning sickness during the first trimester of pregnancy. I believe you are referring to *gond ke laddu* which are traditionally eaten after delivery and not during pregnancy. There are two types of *ladoos*, both are very good and tasty but are very fattening. So eat just one or two every day and remember to have a big glass of milk with it.

Pollutants and their effects

59. What are the effects of pollution on pregnancy?

Q. **How does pollution affect pregnancy? Can it be fatal?**

A. Environmental pollution can be in the air we breathe, the water we drink, the surfaces (e.g. table) we touch, and the food (contaminated food) we eat. Pollutants can be infectious organisms, e.g. neonatal nurses and nursery teachers are exposed to cytomegalovirus, daycare workers are exposed to rubella and parvoviruses, doctors are exposed to tubercle bacilli through droplets, and anyone can be exposed to typhoid bacilli and hepatitis A virus through contaminated water and food. They can have severe effects on the fetus (baby) and the mother. Pregnant industrial workers can be exposed to heavy metals and solvents. Women working in the fields can be exposed to harmful chemicals through pesticides and contaminated well water. Tobacco smoke and high levels of carbon monoxide are common pollutants at the work place and streets with heavy vehicular traffic. The effect of noise pollution on the fetus has not been well-researched. There is scant knowledge regarding the effects of the majority of the chemical pollutants that a pregnant woman can be exposed to in the house, fields or industry. It is believed that an adult's safe level of chemical exposure is 5–10 times higher than the level of fetal tolerance. All women who are pregnant as such should be very careful regarding environmental pollution; they should preferably take care before planning a pregnancy.

Lead is known to be associated with abortion, preterm labour, stillbirth and pregnancy-induced hypertension. It is used in industries such as printing, smelting, batteries and paints. It is an occupational hazard for women working in these industries. Lead pipes are no longer used in most places for water. Organic solvents such as spirits, varnish, kerosene, benzene and acetone are associated with low birth weight in rats when they are exposed to these chemicals for a long time. Some chemicals used as pesticides, insecticides and fungicides can result in an adverse outcome if consumed along with foods. Air pollution with methyl isocyanate (MIC) during the Bhopal gas tragedy (in 1984) markedly increased the incidence of abortion, low birth-weight babies, and stillbirths. In India, we need to have legislation defining safety levels of chemicals for industrial workers and agriculturists.

Even though pollution may be bad, it is not as much a risk to the unborn child as you might think. There have been millions of healthy babies born in major cities without any apparent increased risk from air pollution. Still, precautions may be advisable in certain conditions and here are some ways that you can cut down your intake of unhealthy air.

Avoid smoke-filled rooms. Keep the air-conditioning on in your car, if you are fortunate enough to have the facility, when in congested traffic. Care should also be exercised when using household products. If a product has a strong odour or fumes, do not inhale it directly, or better still, don't use it. Try to avoid using insecticides. Stay away from paint removers and paint fumes.

60. What impact can environmental pollution have on the fetus?

Q. **Will environmental pollution affect my unborn child?**

A. Environmental pollution is a fact of life in cities, towns and villages, but there is no evidence that pregnancies in deserts, clear mountains, etc. - areas away from pollution - lead to any advantage. Some common pollutants that harm babies are smoking and certain drugs. The risk of other pollutants is individual and depends on proximity and factors such as the duration of exposure. Each case is individual, but pollution in general, by definition, is not healthy at any time, perhaps more so when immunity may be lower as a result of pregnancy.

61. Are petrol and pesticide fumes harmful if inhaled during pregnancy?

Q. **I was exposed to petrol (benzene) as it was poured in the house to control**

insects. My 2-year-old daughter was with me too. Was it safe for her? I was pregnant and became a bit dizzy for a few minutes, is that normal? I was also exposed to pesticide fumes in early pregnancy. Could it have any effect on the fetus? My house was painted and paint fumes remained in the house for several days. I was also exposed to paint remover fumes, which came from an open container. It had a very strong smell. Will it have any effect on the pregnancy or on my daughter?

A. Spray from petrol and pesticides is usually inhaled in very small amounts and, at the most, will precipitate allergic cough in your daughter. Regarding your pregnancy, which appears to be of 4 weeks' duration at the time of exposure, it should not be affected by inhalation of sprays, unless these are consumed orally, which may be toxic. If the exposure has been at around 4 weeks of pregnancy and the pregnancy has survived, that means the fetus has most likely escaped the toxic effects, if there were any.

62. Is passive smoking during pregnancy harmful?

Q. In my office my bosses and other staff smoke a lot and the smell of the smoke upsets me. I plan to have a baby and I want to know whether this will affect my pregnancy. I do not smoke myself. Should I leave the job due to this?

A. Smoking, both active as well as passive (as in your case), is bad for the health of everybody. For a pregnant lady it can lead to some problems such as a small, underweight baby, a slight increase in the chances of a miscarriage, etc. It is best to avoid it as far as possible. However, in our society, it is not always possible to achieve this in totality. After all, it is not possible to change the environment in a short period of time.

I would advise you not to leave the job if you need to work. Try and gently counsel your bosses. Keep your table at a location where the smoke has the least chance of reaching in high concentration. You may also ask for the creation of certain 'smoking areas' where smokers can go and smoke so that passive smoking is not a problem for non-smokers. Changing your job is no guarantee that you will find a healthier environment. If you do not need to work, you may of course quit your job so that you undergo your pregnancy in a smoke-free environment. During pregnancy, eat well and look after your nutrition very well and stay under the care of an obstetrician. Also, if your husband smokes, he too should stop smoking. (*See also* page 13)

63. What is the effect of smoking during pregnancy?

Q. **I gave birth to a beautiful and normal child 3-and-a-half years back. Now, I am pregnant for the second time. I have been smoking for the past 2 years, an average of 2 cigarettes a day. I did not know I was pregnant the first month and I was smoking about 4 a day. I am off it now, but I had been smoking for the first 20 days of conception. Will this harm my baby? I need to know this. This is almost the end of my 3rd month.**

A. Cigarette smoking in general, is not good in pregnancy. If you have completely quit now, the baby should be fine. As you have smoked a small number so far, I don't see that any major damage has been done. Please try not to pick up cigarettes again, even after the baby is born. Kids raised in smoking households tend to get more infections, colds and other problems.

Cigarette smoke contains a number of potential teratogens (substances that cause malformations in the baby). Smoking has a direct dose–response effect on fetal (unborn baby) growth. Women who stop smoking early in pregnancy generally have babies with normal birth weights. Smoking during pregnancy is associated with an increased incidence of abortion, preterm labour, low-lying placenta (placenta praevia) and premature separation of the placenta (abruptio placentae) with bleeding during pregnancy. Smoking is associated with an increased incidence of a congenital defect sequence caused by an interruption of blood supply to the chest and arm of the developing baby. Smoking is also associated with a very high risk of cleft lip and cleft palate in babies born to women with an uncommon defect in the gene for transforming growth factor-alpha. (*See also* pages 13, 145)

64. Can soot and other pollutants have an adverse effect on the fetus?

Q. **I am 5 months pregnant and stay in a region where there are a number of industries in the neighbourhood. My question is whether the soot and smoke from industries will have any bad effect on the baby?**

A. Soot and other types of air pollutants may not only affect animals and people, but developing fetuses too. Recent research has found that genetic mutations caused by some pollutants can be passed through sperm to fetal mice. Presumably, the same thing could happen to human beings. The study identifies airborne particulate matter as a contributor to genetic modifications in mice; however, a direct link between genetic mutations and health effects has not yet been established.

65. Can ethanol inhalation affect my fetus?

Q. I am 6 weeks pregnant and am exposed to alcohol vapour (ethanol) in the laboratory for 5–10 minutes. What are the chances of abnormalities in the fetus due to this?

A. I do not feel there is any cause for you to worry. Inhalation of high concentrations would have caused central nervous system effects in you, characterized by nausea, headache, dizziness and unconsciousness and may cause respiratory tract irritation. Toxic levels are about 1000 ppm TWA (time-weighted average) or 1900 mg/cmm TWA.

Fetal alcohol syndrome is seen in babies of alcoholic women who drink heavily and chronically during pregnancy. This results in a distinct pattern of congenital malformations that includes intrauterine and postnatal growth deficiency, a distinctive pattern of physical malformation, and behavioural/cognitive impairment such as fine motor dysfunction and mental retardation. Not all affected children have all the features of the syndrome.

Every laboratory has certain set standards regarding environmental safety for the staff. It is best for you to check with the laboratory in-charge regarding the risks involved in continuing to work during pregnancy. (*See also* page 13)

66. What are the health hazards of inhaling industrial chemicals?

Q. I was exposed to uncovered paint thinner (remover) due to which I had irritation in my nose and throat. I had inhaled it unintentionally from very close. Was it safe for the fetus when I was 6 months pregnant?

A. Industrial chemicals such as paint thinners or paint removers should all be regarded as potentially hazardous. The important issues here are dosage, repetitive exposure, individual susceptibility and special considerations such as pregnancy, genetic or inherited risks, and any additional exposure to interactive or synergistic chemicals or foodstuffs.

All inhalational exposure to industrial or household chemicals can cause temporary airway irritation and some people will develop more severe or prolonged complications such as asthma. Paint thinner may cause dizziness and headache, but if the exposure is limited as in your case, rather than prolonged or repetitive, the symptoms are temporary and no long-term outcome is likely, such as lung or skin damage. In any case, susceptible people should avoid exposure since the long-term effects on pregnancy or the risk of malignancy are unknown, although evidence for such possible detrimental complications is not available in reliable studies.

The potential hazards of all industrial solvents, volatile chemicals and other agents are of general concern. Direct exposure should be minimized or careful precautions such as adequate ventilation should be assured. Potential hazards, including fires, explosions and other risks in addition to their effects on health, necessitate careful handling and very careful disposal. In fact, the appropriate disposal of industrial wastes poses a major environmental risk and all individuals as well as industries should avoid polluting the general atmosphere and water supply. A short and single exposure is unlikely to affect the baby.

67. Are fumes of xylene harmful for the fetus?

Q. I work in a high-volume clinical lab, where there are a lot of fumes of xylene and I am 4 weeks pregnant. My manager tells me that I shouldn't worry, but I am very concerned. Please advise.

A. Xylene (dimethylbenzene or xylol) is an aromatic hydrocarbon solvent commonly found in paints and laboratories. It enters the body rapidly on inhaling and can also be absorbed through the skin, particularly if the period of contact is lengthy. Overexposure to xylene most commonly affects the nervous system, respiratory system and skin. Depending on the levels, it may lead to nausea, headache, feeling high, dizziness, weakness, irritability, vomiting, slowed reaction time, giddiness, confusion, clumsiness, slurred speech, loss of balance, ringing in the ears, etc. Levels greater than 10,000 ppm, may lead to sleepiness, loss of consciousness or even death. The fumes can irritate the eyes, nose and throat while frequent or prolonged skin contact can cause dermatitis with dryness, flaking and cracking of the skin. When the xylene level is >200 ppm, it irritates the lungs causing chest pain and shortness of breath. Extreme overexposure can result in lung oedema.

Studies in pregnant animals have been inconclusive as to whether exposure to very large amounts of xylene (not normally encountered) affect the developing fetus. Extreme levels of xylene that killed some of the pregnant animals caused birth defects in the offspring of the survivors. However, it is still not clear if xylene can affect pregnancy or reproductive function in humans. Common sense demands that pregnant and nursing women minimize their exposure to xylene, just as they should minimize their exposure to alcohol, tobacco and other drugs.

Immunization and investigations

68. What is the immunization and ultrasound schedule during pregnancy?

Q. My wife is pregnant (completed 5 months). (i) Please let us know the names and number of injections to be taken during pregnancy and their dosage schedule. (ii) Also tell us about the ultrasound test and when it should be done. Does it have any effect on the baby?

A. Immunization against tetanus is given in the 6th and 7th months of pregnancy. No other injections are specified in a normal pregnancy. The obstetrician decides, on a case-to-case basis, if any are needed.

Usually three ultrasound scans are done: one in early pregnancy to see the viability of the foetus; the second one at 16–22 weeks to exclude any congenital malformation in the baby; and the third after 8 months of pregnancy to see the proper growth of the baby. However, more ultrasound examinations may be required in specific cases and the obstetrician will decide on that.

There is tremendous controversy whether or not all pregnant women should undergo routine ultrasound screening. The advantages of routine screening include correct dating of pregnancy and early detection of ectopic pregnancy, uterine anomalies and tumours in the ovaries (if done in early pregnancy), ruling out congenital malformations in the baby, early detection of twins and growth problems in the fetus. The Government of India does not include routine ultrasound screening of women at low risk for complications.

Needless to say, the advantages of routine ultrasound screening are directly related to the skill and experience of the ultrasonologist. It has no harmful effect on the baby or the mother.

69. Are vaccines for influenza, hepatitis A and typhoid safe during pregnancy?

Q. I am 25 years old and 7 months pregnant. I am working for a vaccine company. We are into developing human vaccines and I am in the R&D department. As a protective measure all of us are given vaccines such as hepatitis A, *Salmonella typhi*, Hib (*Haemophilius influenzae* b), etc. My doctor has asked me not to take any vaccines during pregnancy. I had a scan after 5 months and the doctor says that everything is fine and there is nothing to worry. I am still working in my lab. I am exposed (if not directly) indirectly to all these antigens. Will the baby inside me have any problems because of this? Are there any tests that I can undergo to know that my baby is fine? I am very tense and worried about my baby. If not now, will the baby in future have any health problems? Please help.

A. Please note that what your doctor said regarding not taking these vaccines during pregnancy is correct.

Most importantly, the director of the R&D lab where you are currently working would know the risks involved (if any) of posting a pregnant woman in such a lab. I am sure your immediate superior and boss are aware that you are pregnant. Every lab has strict guidelines laid down as far as professional hazards are concerned so that employees are not exposed to these risks. The best thing for you to do is to discuss these matters with the director of your lab immediately.

Hepatitis A is caused mainly by intake of contaminated food or water, and at times through sexual contact with a person with hepatitis A. The virus does not cause malformations in the unborn baby. Risk of transmission to the unborn baby is negligible; the baby can get infected during vaginal delivery. Severe infection with hepatitis A virus during pregnancy can result in preterm labour and sometimes in death of the baby and the mother. These adverse outcomes are more commonly noted in women who are poorly nourished and who develop severe hepatitis. The pregnant woman recently exposed by close personal or sexual contact to a person with hepatitis A should receive prophylaxis with immunoglobulin. Inactivated virus vaccine can be administered to a pregnant woman, if there is a risk of contracting the infection. Two doses are administered, with the second dose given 6–12 months after the first.

Typhoid is caused by intake of contaminated food, water or milk. Severe infection can result in abortion, preterm labour and death of the newborn and the mother. Typhoid vaccine does not seem to exert any harmful effect when administered to a pregnant woman. It is a live attenuated bacterial vaccine (Ty21a), and therefore, one should consider the risks versus the benefits before administering the vaccine to pregnant women. It is recommended that pregnant women should be vaccinated with the typhoid vaccine during an epidemic or before travel to an endemic area.

Infection with *Haemophilus influenzae* results in lung infection (pneumonitis). Prompt diagnosis is the key to avoid adverse effects. The frequency of preterm labour is slightly increased. With prompt treatment with antibiotics, there are very few deaths among babies and mothers, and occur only in severe cases requiring treatment in intensive care units (ICU). There are no efficacy data to recommend the use of Hib vaccine to adults with an increased risk for Hib.

70. What vaccinations are required during pregnancy?

Q. Presently my wife is pregnant. During pregnancy women usually take three vaccinations. What are these and when are they given?

A. The Government of India recommends that all pregnant women be immunized with two injections of tetanus toxoid at 20 weeks and 25 weeks, respectively. No other vaccines are routinely recommended.

71. Is a tetanus toxoid shot necessary during pregnancy?

Q. My wife is 6 months pregnant. She has taken TT Tetvac injection, advised by the doctor. The doctor told us that she should take another injection next month. Is TT Tetvac essential during pregnancy?

A. Immunization of the pregnant woman leads to protection of the baby from tetanus during delivery. This occurs by transfer of antibodies from the mother to the unborn baby through the placenta. Tetanus is a major cause of death among newborns in developing countries. It occurs when delivery occurs in unhygienic places, and the baby acquires it when the umbilical cord is cut by a contaminated blade or pair of scissors after delivery. As tetanus toxoid does not cause adverse effects in the pregnant woman, it is given to all pregnant women, irrespective of where she will deliver. The first dose can be administered any time after 14 weeks of pregnancy and the second dose 1 month later. If a woman has never received primary tetanus immunization or the history of complete primary immunization is uncertain, she should receive a third injection of the toxoid 6–12 months after the second dose. Subsequently, she needs to have 1 booster injection every 10 years.

The pregnant woman needs to have only 1 injection of the toxoid if the primary immunization was complete and the last booster dose was received within the past 10 years. Most Indian women do not take the third dose of the primary immunization and have uncertain histories of immunization; therefore, the Government of India recommends at least two injections of tetanus toxoid during pregnancy.

72. Is the administration of Rabipur vaccine safe during pregnancy?

Q. A mouse had bitten my wife. She is 6 weeks pregnant. The doctor administered Rabipur vaccine to her. Is it safe? Should she go for the second dose?

A. Rabipur vaccine is safe. Because of the potential consequences of untreated rabies exposure and because rabies vaccination has not been associated with fetal abnormalities, anti-rabies vaccination is allowed during pregnancy.

It is best to administer the rabies immunoglobulin immediately after the bite along with the vaccine.

73. How safe is varicella vaccination during pregnancy?

Q. I found out that I was 3 weeks pregnant a week after receiving a varicella vaccination. What are the chances of abnormalities in the foetus and pregnancy due to this? Is terminating the pregnancy recommended?

A. The manufacturers of varicella vaccine and drug control authorities recommend that (a) it should not be given to women who are expecting, and (b) non-pregnant women should use contraception for three months after injection. These recommendations are given to avoid malpractice suits in case something goes wrong. Scientifically no studies have been conducted to determine the effect of the vaccine on the unborn baby. Such a trial cannot be done because of ethical reasons. Thus, we do not really know whether the vaccine has an adverse effect or not. The vaccine is a live attenuated virus vaccine and the virus can infect the unborn baby with the highest risk between 13 and 20 weeks. Women should not get pregnant for a minimum of 1 month after being vaccinated. Merck & Co. has established a registry to follow outcomes when women are vaccinated within 3 months before becoming pregnant or at any time during pregnancy. Even though the risk of infection in the unborn baby is very small (less than 2%) and theoretical, the decision is finally left to the pregnant woman. One case has been reported where a pregnant woman got infected from the vaccine strain of varicella from her child. As an abundant precaution, the pregnancy was terminated. However, when the fetus was tested, there was no sign of varicella infection. Thus, in retrospect, the termination of pregnancy was not required.

In your case, you were 2 weeks pregnant at the time of vaccination. Though this is not the period of greatest risk, the decision is ultimately yours. Whatever you do, please remember that ultrasound cannot detect all abnormalities.

Illness and pregnancy

74. Why do I feel weak and dizzy during my pregnancy?

Q. I have just entered my 8th month of pregnancy. My blood pressure since the beginning of the pregnancy has been around 90/60 mmHg, which, I understand, is on the lower side. I have gained only 5 kg since the start of the pregnancy. My doctor was initially concerned about the BP and low weight but felt that as long as I was feeling all right with no signs of tiredness or fatigue, this could be the normal range for me. I have had no problems till now and consider myself fairly active with a 10-hour job and a young child at home. I wish to continue to work till the last day and remain active. For the past two days, I have been feeling slightly dizzy and thought it may be because of the summer heat, though I continue to take fluids and try to eat every 3–4 hours. Please advise if I need to take any further precautions.

A. I think the 10 hours of work every day and looking after a small child when you are pregnant are too much for you. That is one reason you are feeling dizzy. The summer heat is an additional factor. Hope you do not have a tendency for diabetes (please check your family history). I also suppose your doctor has made sure your baby is growing satisfactorily.

This is the time that the baby grows maximally (in terms of weight). A small-for-date baby can face lots of problems before, during and after birth.

In view of this and your workload, I feel you should go on maternity leave right away, since there is no need to continue working when it is already causing undue fatigue.

You are paying a big premium to have a healthy baby – end result should be good for both the baby and you. Adequate rest and sleep along with a good diet will help you and your baby. Keep away from the heat outside. If your house gets hot, install an air conditioner (if possible) or a cooler. Drink lots of fluids - tender coconut water, barley lime water, glucose-D with a dash of lime and salt, etc.

75. How is migraine treated during pregnancy?

Q. My 29-year-old wife is 5 months pregnant. This is her first pregnancy and she suffers from migraine. My family doctor started treating her headache with Flunarine tablets but discontinued after the pregnancy was detected. Now she gets repeated attacks that we control with Crocin (paracetamol). Can these attacks by themselves harm the baby in any way? What is the best way to treat them?

A. Congratulations on the pregnancy! Migraine headaches can get better or worse during a pregnancy. Unfortunately, your wife falls in the latter category. Migraine headaches themselves are not known to have adverse effects on the baby. In general, physicians only use medicines that are safe in pregnancy. Any pain product based on acetaminophen is relatively safe. Combining this with an anti-nausea medicine such as Phenergan is sometimes very effective in stopping migraine headaches. Ergotamine, which is very effective in treating migraines, should not be used during pregnancy. Sumatriptan, which is also effective in treating migraine, has been found to be harmful to embryos in animals. It has not been studied extensively in pregnant women. Your wife can be treated with propranolol, atenolol or amitryptiline.

There is some evidence that calcium and magnesium supplements can prevent migraine attacks. The most important thing to do is to identify and avoid the triggers.

It is important to note that migraine symptoms are similar to those of other more serious disorders. Hence, a complete evaluation by a neurologist and neuroimaging studies should be performed, if necessary.

76. Will a low haemoglobin affect my pregnancy?

Q. I am in the 8th month of my pregnancy. After a blood test I got to know that my haemoglobin is low – it is only 8 g/dl. My doctor has asked me to take injections to increase my haemoglobin level. But when I took the second dose I had a complete blackout. I was sweating but I have to take 10 such injections. Will a low haemoglobin affect my pregnancy? Can you

please help me? I also sweat and feel stressed and weak. How do I increase my haemoglobin?

A. About 80% of Indian women are anaemic, i.e. have haemoglobin less than 12 g/dl (<11 g/dl for pregnant women) with the usual cause being physiological loss of blood during the menstrual cycle combined with inadequate nutritional intake. The problem gets compounded in pregnancy when the body's need for iron goes up. Anaemia during pregnancy may cause problems for both the baby and mother, and that is why every pregnant lady is prescribed iron and folic acid tablets. Anaemic women are prone to infections (especially urinary tract infections), preterm labour, pre-eclampsia, and collapse even with normal blood loss during delivery. The baby can be small for date and preterm in women with severe anaemia, or even die *in utero*. A haemoglobin level less than 7 g/dl is considered severe, between 7 and 9 g/dl moderate and above 9 and less than 11 g/dl mild.

Iron dextran injections (Imferon) are administered intramuscularly over a period of time (depending upon the total calculated dose required). However, allergy to the drug can occur with 'blackouts and sweating'. I suspect this is what you underwent. Your other symptoms are due to the anaemia. As the rate of rise of haemoglobin on taking iron tablet or injection is the same, you can also take oral iron tablets but make sure that 100 mg of elemental iron per day is taken, preferably along with fruit juice. An iron-rich diet (meat, eggs, green vegetables, etc.) is a must. Please consult your doctor to clarify which injection you received and the need for it.

It is also important to establish the cause of anaemia, ensure a good balanced diet, and rule out other nutritional deficiencies. Worm infestation, attacks of malaria in the recent past, urinary tract infection, bleeding piles, gastric ulcers and thalassaemia trait need to be ruled out.

77. What is the cure for rashes near the vagina during pregnancy?

Q. I am 4 months pregnant. I take progesterone 200 and folic acid. Are these all right? I have a very serious problem of allergy and rashes near my vagina. I had applied niycle, rashfree, coconut oil and a lot of other things but day by day my allergy and itching is only increasing. I am not comfortable even while sitting. And right now that portion is totally dry and appears whitish.

A. You most likely have candidal vulvovaginitis. The diagnosis can be confirmed by clinical examination and potassium hydroxide (KOH)/saline examination of vaginal discharge demonstrating budding yeast cells of *Candida* in it. The treatment in a pregnant women for this condition is clotrimazole vaginal tablet (100 mg) (available as Candid vaginal tablet), one tablet at night inserted deep intravaginally with an applicator for 5 days or so. On the sore skin outside, one can use clotrimazole (Candid cream, Canstat cream) or any other azole (miconazole, ketoconazole) cream twice daily topically. Orally, an antihistamine tablet like Avil (chlorpheniramine) can be safely taken daily at night to control the itching. Oral antifungals (fluconazole, ketoconazole, or itraconazole) are best avoided in the early pregnancy. Consult a dermatologist for further details.

78. Does low blood pressure affect pregnancy in any way?

Q. **I am 26 years old and married for 2-and-a-half years. I currently live in the US. I will be back in India early next year. Recently, I had a general check-up here and they said my BP is slightly on the lower side, around 90/60 mmHg. We are trying for a baby now. Would this low blood pressure affect my pregnancy in any way? How do I bring it back to normal? Do I have to take any medication?**

A. Blood pressure of 90/60 mmHg is not a disease. If you have no other problem, this is in fact a very good blood pressure to keep heart attacks, strokes and all vascular problems away.

Lower blood pressures in healthy people are welcome as per guidelines and epidemiological studies. Pregnancy should be no problem. You may like to get a general examination done by your doctor.

79. How can one manage pregnancy-induced hypertension? Is aspirin harmful in pregnancy?

Q. **My wife is 27 years old. The first pregnancy ended in intrauterine death (IUD) (abruptio placentae due to high BP) at the 25th week. The BP was found to be normal during the earlier check-ups. It was also found that there was excess protein in the urine, which became normal after delivery. The BP became normal after 3 months with medication, which was stopped thereafter. Six months later she conceived again. The doctor prescribed**

aspirin (delayed release, 75 mg per day) this time from the first month onwards. However, this too ended in a missed abortion during the 10th week. As a follow-up, blood antibodies were checked and were normal. The reason for these miscarriages is not known. Could aspirin have caused this? What are the risks of taking aspirin? Should it be taken again in the next pregnancy? Are these two miscarriages related? Will they recur and what precautions are needed the next time?

A. Pregnancy-induced hypertension, especially if associated with protein in the urine (proteinuria), can be a cause of intrauterine death and placental abruption. However, one would think that 25 weeks is a bit too early to have a complication like that, especially if the rise in blood pressure was mild to moderate. On the other hand, if it has happened in the first pregnancy, she is certainly more likely to have high blood pressure in the later pregnancies, though they may be less harmful for the pregnancy next time. By and large, pregnancy-induced hypertension gets better with each pregnancy.

Of course, there are no hard and fast rules in medicine, and the reverse may be true in some cases. The role of aspirin in pregnancy-induced hypertension is controversial. It is certainly not indispensable. Aspirin has recently been reported to be associated with a high risk of earlier abortions, and so your concern is justified. The exact risk in an individual case is difficult to determine, as early abortions are common anyway. Whether your wife needs aspirin in the next pregnancy will have to be decided by the treating physician. Once your wife is pregnant again, you would have to take the decision right then.

Needless to say, aspirin is not the end all of management of hypertension in pregnancy. In fact, due to its complicated mode of action it may actually be associated with a higher risk of early abortions and placental abruption. Certainly there is no need to give aspirin in the first few months of pregnancy. Once a live pregnancy is established by ultrasound examination, after the 16th week or so, you can consider using low-dose aspirin, and that too only if the blood flow seems to be less than adequate. However, if you choose not to use aspirin at all, I can assure you that it would not harm the pregnancy in any way. The role of aspirin in these cases has only been speculated on and has not yet been proven beyond doubt.

As far as precautions are concerned, you can keep a close watch on the blood pressure and the amount of protein in the urine during the next pregnancy. You may need to monitor the blood flow through the placental and fetal vessels by Doppler studies. No specific precautions such as avoiding travel and work are required. In fact, she should lead as normal a life as possible. This will give her more confidence and increase the chances of having a normal pregnancy. In case she develops hypertension in the next pregnancy or passes protein in the urine she would require treatment for blood pressure. The pregnancy must be looked after by an expert trained to look after high-risk pregnancies.

There is nothing to suggest that the two pregnancy losses are related to each other in any way. Early abortions generally occur when the fetus itself is less than perfectly formed. Nature does not preserve abnormal fetuses and this leads to an early abortion, while placental abruption and hypertension occur during late pregnancy and are worse in the first pregnancy. Subsequently the risk of developing hypertension is there but is generally a milder type and causes less damage to the fetus. To completely answer your question as to whether the two miscarriages were related, one would have to do a few tests on your wife to find out what went wrong. She would require a complete work-up with a complete blood count, blood sugar to rule out diabetes, check the kidney functions, exclude infections and exclude antiphospholipid syndrome (APLS) by doing lupus anticoagulant and anticardiolipin tests. If all these tests do not reveal any abnormalities, one can safely presume that the two abortions were because of independent reasons and she should go ahead in a positive frame of mind and plan the next pregnancy. I wish you all the luck for the next pregnancy.

80. What are the effects of sickle cell anaemia during pregnancy?

Q. I want to know in detail about the effects of sickle cell anaemia during pregnancy and its possible treatment.

A. Till recently, pregnancy was discouraged in patients with sickle cell disease, as such women are at an increased risk for vaso-occlusive crisis, pregnancy induced hypertension, pyelonephritis, thrombophlebitis, and spontaneous abortion compared with the general population. Hypertension is the most common complication during such pregnancies and nearly 20% of pregnancies may result in preterm deliveries and infants that are small for gestational age.

Close monitoring, prompt diagnosis and aggressive treatment of complications during the prenatal and neonatal period is important.

Prenatal care requires a team (obstetrician, physician, haematologist and nutritionist) and patients may require prophylactic transfusion and folic acid supplements to decrease the incidence of vaso-occlusive crisis.

Maternal deaths in women with sickle cell anaemia are low these days, and are reported to vary from 2% to 9% in different centres. One common danger is that symptomatic women may be considered to be suffering from a sickle-cell crisis, and other more serious conditions requiring prompt treatment may be overlooked (e.g. ectopic pregnancy, acute appendicitis, placental abruption, pyelonephritis, etc). The diagnosis of sickle-cell crisis should be made only after ruling out other conditions causing pain or fever, or reduction of haemoglobin.

Almost all women with sickle-cell disease have some cardiac dysfunction; hence these women should be treated like patients with cardiac disease during labour and delivery.

Combined regimens that increase haemoglobin F seem to be promising. Hydroxyurea and 5-azacytidine and recombinant erythropoietin with hydroxyurea have been used. Hydroxyurea decreases crisis attacks by 50%. Hydroxyurea is teratogenic in animals; its experience during human pregnancy is limited. A promising treatment is bone marrow transplantation. Prenatal diagnosis is possible by amniocentesis or chorionic villus sampling. Elective abortion can be performed if the diagnosis is established. Stem cell therapy is a promising alternative treatment *in utero*.

Sickle-cell trait is not a contraindication to pregnancy on the basis of causing increased risk to the mother. However, if the father is a carrier of the gene for abnormal haemoglobin or thalassaemia, there is a 25% chance of the baby suffering from sickle-cell haemoglobinopathy. Prenatal testing is a must in these women.

You need to discuss all the details with your obstetrician.

81. How should low platelet counts be managed during pregnancy?

Q. I am 36 weeks pregnant. I have gestational diabetes and take insulin 4-6-15 units with an 1800-calorie diabetic diet. My platelet count was low (approximately 1 lakh) a month earlier. From the last month, it has reduced further to 60,000–70,000. My nose bleeds every other day. I occasionally feel tired and dizzy also. I am taking Ferrium XT (100 mg) daily. My doctor says that platelet transfusion will be given during labour, if required. What

food should I take to increase the platelet count? Is a count of 60,000 or below serious?

A. The platelet count usually falls as pregnancy progresses, the lowest levels being during the third trimester. Current guidelines recommend that asymptomatic patients with a platelet count of more than 20,000/ml do not require treatment until delivery. Platelet counts of more than 50,000/ml (with a normal coagulation profile) are safe for normal vaginal delivery as also a caesarean section. However, for the use of epidural anaesthesia, the platelet count should be more than 80,000/ml.

Thrombocytopenia (or low platelet count) seen in pregnancy is usually caused by 'gestational thrombocytopenia' (GT), which has no significant bleeding risk to the mother or baby. However, it is difficult to distinguish this condition from 'idiopathic thrombocytopenia (ITP)', in which antibodies develop against one's own platelets. These antibodies can cross the placenta and cause bleeding in the fetus or newborn.

Low platelet count during pregnancy may also be due to some complication of pregnancy such as pre-eclampsia, or secondary to some underlying disease. Thus, you should be examined and tested to exclude pre-eclampsia; disseminated intravascular coagulation; haemolytic uraemic syndrome/thrombotic thrombocytopenic purpura; autoimmune thrombocytopenia – idiopathic/drug-related/systemic lupus erythematosus (SLE)/antiphospholipid syndrome/infection-related; folate deficiency; coincidental marrow disease and hypersplenism.

Treatment is with corticosteroids or intravenous gammaglobulins. Steroids are used if the duration of treatment is likely to be short, i.e. starting in the third trimester. Prolonged steroid therapy may cause significant side-effects and in such cases intravenous gammaglobulin therapy should be considered. If there is no response to oral steroids or intravenous gammaglobulins, high-dose intravenous methyl prednisolone alone or in combination with intravenous gammaglobulins or treatment with azathioprine is indicated. Splenectomy is an effective treatment in women who do not respond to steroids or immunoglobulin therapy. However, this operation can be difficult late in pregnancy, and may need to be combined with an elective caesarean section.

Platelet infusion should be administered for life-threatening haemorrhage and be available prior to surgery for patients with severe thrombocytopenia. However, a platelet transfusion alone is of no use in the case of ITP, as the transfused platelets would be destroyed.

Thrombocytopenia in the newborn can occur in those babies born to women with thrombocytopenia, especially those suffering from ITP not related to pregnancy, however, the risks of clinically dangerous thrombocytopenia in newborns is very low.

Because of the low incidence of neonatal thrombocytopenia, most obstetricians do not perform cordocentesis (aspirating umbilical cord blood when the baby is still inside the uterus) to avoid the risks involved. Scalp blood testing for fetal monitoring in labour should be avoided. Caesarean section to prevent intracranial haemorrhage in the newborn is controversial. The cord blood should definitely be collected at the time of delivery to rule out thrombocytopenia in the newborn. All women with thrombocytopenia must deliver in a hospital that has adequate blood and blood components and a neonatal ICU.

There is no diet that affects the platelet count. Continue to take iron and folic acid.

82. What are the causes for a positive ANA test during pregnancy?

Q. I am 28 weeks pregnant with my second child. My blood type is B negative. I have received Rhogam four times in my lifetime, once after a miscarriage (at six weeks), once during my first pregnancy, after the birth of my first child and about one-and-a-half weeks ago for this pregnancy. At my last check-up, the doctor performed the usual dipstick test and found protein in my urine. She asked me to do a 24-hour urine test, which showed a level of 455. I don't have high blood pressure, my creatine levels are normal and my complete blood count (CBC) was normal. My obstetrician then referred me to a nephrologist. The nephrologist told me to undergo an ANA test, which was positive. All the other work-up done for the kidney function panel was normal. The nephrologist told me to go for a lupus test, even though the only symptom of lupus that I have is protein in my urine. Is Anti-D, the substance in the Rhogam shots, considered an antinuclear antibody? If so, would it cause my ANA test to be falsely positive?

A. Antinuclear antibodies (ANA) are an unusual type of gamma-globulins found in patients with certain autoimmune diseases. ANA are directed against certain components found in the nucleus of a cell in the body. They are found in patients whose immune system is predisposed to cause inflammation against their own body tissues (autoimmune diseases).

An ANA test is needed if there is a reasonable suspicion of systemic lupus erythematosus (SLE) from the history, physical findings or the results of routine tests such as the CBC (leukopenia, thrombocytopenia) as ANA may be found in a variety of conditions and in normal individuals. The random chance of a false positive in normal individuals is considerably greater than a true positive, unless the clinician selects only individuals with a reasonably high possibility of having the disease before testing. Even with the newest tests, about 5% (1 out of 20) of normal individuals will give a weakly positive result and ANA should never be ordered as a routine screening test. A positive ANA result in a patient with no or minimal features of SLE can be misleading or worse because it may cause the clinician to order unnecessary tests.

It is possible that anti-D is non-specifically binding and causing a false positive test result. You can go for immunofluorescence-based tests in case ANA is positive with ELISA.

83. Could stomach ache during pregnancy be serious?

Q. I am 2 months pregnant and suffer from moderate stomach ache throughout the day. Please advise.

A. It is difficult to diagnose the cause of your stomach ache without personally examining you. It could be a simple case of gastritis (take a bland diet, avoid spicy food, take Gelusil MPS, 2 tablets to be chewed after meals). Another common cause is colitis. If you do not have urinary symptoms, it cannot be urinary tract infection. I suggest you report this to your gynaecologist immediately, for a thorough evaluation.

84. What can safely be taken for dry cough during pregnancy?

Q. I am 22 weeks pregnant and have been suffering from sinusitis and dry cough for the past week. I have severe bouts of cough. I am worried as to whether the baby will be harmed due to my coughing. My doctor has suggested I use Linctus Codeine but when I surfed the net, I found that it isn't very safe for the fetus. I take steam inhalations and gargle, but this is not of much help. What should I do?

A. For dry cough during pregnancy, the best option is to do frequent steam inhalations. You can put Sinarest vapocaps in the water. I hope you are already taking folic acid which is mandatory during pregnancy to prevent malformations in the baby.

85. Can pregnant women undergo LASIK?

Q. **I am 8 months pregnant. I am supposed to undergo a medical examination for a higher post in a quasi-government organization. My eye power is –5.00 and I wear contact lenses for the past 9 years. I understand that the organization might demand –4.00 as a specification. I was planning to undergo LASIK surgery and then take the medical exam. But I am discouraged by the fact that lactating/nursing mothers should not undergo LASIK. What should I do now?**

A. It is not ideal to do LASIK for multiple reasons:

- Poor stability of the refractive power during and after pregnancy
- Unpredictable outcomes of laser treatment due to hormonal influences
- There is a risk of injury to the eye by the child post-operatively
- The medicines used may reach the baby through the breast milk.

I would suggest that you wait for 6 months following delivery.

86. How can hypothyroidism be managed during pregnancy?

Q. **I am in my 7th month of pregnancy. I have hypothyroidism and am taking Eltroxin 100 mcg. My recent thyroid profile shows – FT3 – 1.6 (1.2–4.2 pg/dl); FT4 – 0.6 (0.8–2.0 ng/dl); TSH – 0.9 (0.4–6.0 MIU/ml). My doctor has increased my dosage to 150 mcg. Is it enough? Is my FT4 too low? Will hypothyroidism affect my child? Will my Eltroxin dosage be reduced after delivery?**

A. Women need more thyroid hormone during pregnancy and, unlike normal women, those with hypothyroidism are unable to increase thyroidal thyroxine hormone (T4 and T3) secretion. Women may need higher doses of thyroxine (tablet) during pregnancy; up to 45% more than pre-pregnancy levels.

We recommend more frequent monitoring. The increase in thyroxine dose begins at about week 8 and peaks by week 16 of pregnancy.

After a woman's new optimal T4 dose is established, the frequency of blood monitoring can be decreased to approximately once every trimester. Serum (blood test) thyroid stimulating hormone (TSH) levels should be measured every four weeks until the TSH becomes normal, thereafter it is measured less frequently.

After delivery, a woman's dose of thyroxine will need to be readjusted and most often patients will go back to the pre-pregnancy dose.

Women with hypothyroidism whose thyroxine (T4) levels are carefully regulated during pregnancy (as it seems in your case) have normal children. You will need another test (TSH and FT4) 4 weeks after you have increased the dose of thyroxine and then again 4 weeks after delivery.

87. If a woman is epileptic, can it harm her fetus?

Q. I am 18 weeks pregnant. I have been taking Tegretal (carbamazepine) 200 mg twice a day for the past 3 years, but haven't had any seizures since then. My doctor suggested I take Microgest in my 1st, 2nd and 3rd month. But I read on your site that Microgest is harmful. I take Livogen-Z, Tegretal 200 mg, Cobadex and Macalvit now. I had a triple marker test and carbamazepine level test done, and both results were normal. The ultrasound was fine too. I am scared for the baby's mental health. Please tell me if I should do any more tests or take any other precautions.

A. Since you have had no seizures in the past 3 years, you are in a much better situation to have a baby and after the birth of the baby can gradually stop medication under medical advice.

Unfortunately, there are a lot of misconceptions among lay people about epilepsy. A person with well-controlled epilepsy is as normal as a person without epilepsy.

A majority of women with well-controlled epilepsy (with medication) have a normal pregnancy and normal babies. The frequency of seizures remains the same in 50%, increases in 30% and reduces in 20% of pregnant women. Since you have had no seizures, I think there would be no problem in the remaining period. In the unlikely event of your getting a seizure, the dose of carbamazepine should be increased by about 50%.

Abnormality in children born to mothers on anti-epileptic drugs is 5%–6%. This figure is not that alarming, since even in women without epilepsy, the abnormality figure is about 2%–3%. As another precaution, you can have the alfa-fetoprotein level of the blood measured, if this test is available in the place where you reside.

At the moment you are on the minimal dose of carbamazepine. This must be continued during pregnancy. The risk of withdrawal of medicine is much more than continuation of therapy. In addition, 20 mg daily of vitamin K should be taken in the last 2 weeks of pregnancy and the infant should be given 1 mg of vitamin K on birth to prevent bleeding.

Carbamazepine is excreted in the mother's milk to the extent of 25%–60%; hence the baby should be watched for side-effects such as drowsiness and allergic skin reactions. In your case, an attempt can also be made to gradually stop the medication once the baby is in your lap.

Unless you are suffering from any specific deficiency, there is no need to swallow unnecessary, multi-ingredient vitamin/mineral supplements. What you need is a larger-than-normal dose of folic acid due to the epilepsy and medication.

Livogen-Z contains 0.75 mg folic acid and iron. Cobadex contains B-complex factors, vitamin C and again folic acid 1.5 mg. This quantity of folic acid is not adequate. You should take 5 mg of folic acid till labour. Multi-ingredient products do not contain this quantity of folic acid. Hence, you should take Folet or Folvite, one tablet a day. Both contain 5 mg of folic acid.

If your haemoglobin is low, you can take an iron product such as slow-release Fecontin-Z Continus - a tablet daily. Slow-release iron is preferable since it is easy on the stomach.

It is not necessary to take other supplements. Excessive water-soluble vitamins are thrown out by the body via the kidneys.

Infections

88. What should I do to manage a cold during pregnancy?

Q. I am 5 months pregnant and have a severe cold for the past 15 days. I took Coldact but it doesn't seem to help. What are the possible effects of cold on the baby? Please suggest some remedy.

A. A 'cold' can be incapacitating. Treatment with steam inhalations, paracetamol (Crocin), and vitamin C is usually helpful. Importantly, one should take precautions to avoid catching a cold during pregnancy. Avoid sitting close to people who are suffering from a 'cold', crowded and congested rooms and market places, keep warm during chilly days (winter and rainy seasons), avoid dusting and congested roads while travelling.

It is important to note that Coldact (chlorpheniramine plus phenylpropanolamine), which is usually present with other ingredients in the common tablets used for cold, is found to be associated with a slight increased incidence of minor anomalies like club foot, inguinal hernia, and eye and ear deformities when taken in the first three months of pregnancy. This drug crosses the placenta and blood-brain barrier and causes hyperactivity and increases fetal heart rate, after being taken by the pregnant lady. Therefore, this is best avoided during pregnancy - especially in the first trimester - in women with hypertension, and in those with placental insufficiency and poor fetal growth.

89. Why is the TORCH test done during pregnancy?

Q. I am in my early stages of pregnancy. Recently, I noticed an itchy red rash

on my entire body. I was advised by my doctor to take a dose of Avil (chlorpheniramine) as it could be some allergic reaction. However, the rash did not subside. Subsequently, my gynaecologist asked me to undergo a TORCH test as it could be some viral infection. I have not had the MMR vaccine. The test showed CMV IgM – 0.15 and IgG – 4.10 while Rubella IgM was 0.14 and IgG 28.8. My doctor was quite alarmed but asked me not to worry because if the infection reaches the fetus, it would either stop growing (in which case it would abort by itself) or it would lag in growth by the 9th week, when she advised an ultrasound examination. The repeat TORCH test showed that the CMV levels were more or less the same but the Rubella IgM had gone down to 0.02 and IgG to 9.3. In the 9th week I underwent an ultrasonography and the doctor told me that the growth of the fetus was fine – it measured 24 mm and had a heart rate of 169 per minute. The doctor also suggested that things seemed to be fine but that I should go in for another USG at 13 weeks. In case growth at this stage was also normal, we could safely presume that all was well and go ahead with the pregnancy. Of course, he would also do another ultrasound at 18–20 weeks in the normal course to ascertain all was well. I have a few questions with regard to my case: Rubella is known to cause congenital disorders in children if contracted by the mother in the 1st trimester. Can the level of infection I had have such an effect? The IgM test is supposedly a better indicator of current infection – is it normal to have some antibodies in the reference range or should it be zero? In case the growth of the fetus is normal at 13 weeks, can I safely assume that the virus has not affected the fetus? Is there any other way of testing if an unborn child has some disorder(s), not just physical (which can be seen by ultrasound, I presume), but also mental/neurological disorders? Is it safe to go ahead with the pregnancy if all is well at the 13th week, as I would rather terminate the pregnancy than take any chance of having a crippled child?

A. You have written the details of the tests and the dates, but have not mentioned the reference range used by the lab from where you got the tests done. Each test is to be evaluated against the reference range of the lab written in brackets in the reports given to you. And from the reference points that I use, all these tests for rubella and CMV seem to be within the normal range, so I do not quite understand why you and your doctor are so worried. But you will have to cross-check these tests with the reference range given by the lab that you got the tests done from. If the IgM is less than the reference range you do not have to worry at all.

Rubella is devastating if it infects a mother in the first three months and there is no question of going through with the pregnancy irrespective of the ultrasound reports since the chances of having an abnormal child are very high. Fortunately, there is no evidence to suggest that you had rubella clinically as the rash of rubella lasts only a few hours (maximum up to a day or so) while you had a persistent rash (as apparent from what you wrote) and it seems some kind of a skin condition.

The IgG and IgM reports do not suggest an active infection. And there are some discrepancies in the reports. If the IgG was positive, it will remain positive probably for the rest of your life and it only means that you had the infection, like most of us, sometime in the past in which case you do not have to worry at all. Rubella is a once-in-a-lifetime infection and once you have had it, it will give you life-long immunity. Unless you take steroids or have a serious immune deficiency you cannot have rubella again.

High IgM levels suggest a recent infection but yours seem to be within the normal range. You have written that the IgG for rubella decreased within a week. IgG levels dropped from about 32 to less than ten units. This does not make any sense to me and one of the two reports must be incorrect since IgG does not drop for decades, leave alone within a week or two. Please get these reports interpreted by the lab where these tests were performed, preferably by a clinical microbiologist or a specialist in infectious diseases, if possible. There is also no proof that you recently had CMV infection (also a viral infection).

IgM is a better indicator of current infection and in your case fortunately it seems to be normal. IgM is never zero as it cross-reacts with many other IgMs and other proteins. We have to follow the reference range provided by the lab.

There is no direct relation between an active infection and ultrasound growth and it can, therefore, not be relied upon as the diagnostic criterion either to confirm or refute the diagnosis of rubella. In fact, it gives us no information at all. You cannot take a decision based on the ultrasound report.

The unborn child cannot be tested for infection by ultrasound. If there is a reasonable suspicion of a fetal infection, the only way to check would be to take the blood from the fetus at twenty weeks and analyse it for IgM against rubella and do a PCR (polymerase chain reaction) diagnosis of rubella.

I do understand your anxiety and in your position I would feel exactly the same – that it is better to abort a possibly abnormal child at this stage.

In my opinion since there is no proof that you recently had rubella or

CMV, you should carry your pregnancy without any further doubt.

The ultrasound at 20 weeks and the triple test at 16 weeks should be done as in all pregnancies to exclude abnormality in the baby, and your case is no different.

I wish you all the best for the rest of the pregnancy. (*See also* page 18)

90. Can vaginal infection during pregnancy harm the baby?

Q. I think I am pregnant. My cycle is between 24 and 27 days. It is already 4 days up and I have never had an irregular cycle till date. I tested twice with Pregcard. It was positive but the second line is lighter than the first one. I also have fungal infection for 2 weeks. My doctor told me to use Cando cream inside the vagina but I stopped using it after I realized that I could be pregnant. I still feel itchy but there is no burning sensation while urinating. I must also tell you that last year I had a miscarriage in my 8th month. The doctor said it happened due to high blood pressure. Throughout my 8 months my blood pressure was 120/80; only a week before the miscarriage it went to 130/90. I had even started on a salt-free diet as I had oedema. Coming back to my current problem – if I am pregnant, will my vaginal infection harm the baby? What precautions should I take?

A. Any infection in the vagina or cervix (mouth of uterus) is not good during pregnancy. However, if it is a fungal infection only (as told by your doctor), it will not cause any harm to the baby now. But it needs to be treated, especially as you have problems. At a later stage in pregnancy, vaginal and cervical infections can lead to numerous problems such as preterm birth, premature rupture of membranes, and their consequences, etc. Vaginal fungal infection just before vaginal delivery can infect the baby during her/his passage through the vagina (birth canal). Applying the cream outside the vagina now will help treat the infection outside the vagina, which you seem to have at present.

You must have a serum beta hCG test done and repeat it 48 hours after the first test. The results will give the doctor a good idea of what is happening – are you pregnant at all, is the pregnancy in the uterus or outside (ectopic pregnancy), if it is an intrauterine pregnancy, is it progressing well, etc. However, before this, you must be examined by an experienced obstetrician and have an ultrasound of the pelvis done by a good ultrasonologist who can do transvaginal sonography as well. The clinical examination is very important as the ultrasound findings can be interpreted best by correlating with the clinical findings.

I emphasize that an experienced obstetrician must examine you immediately.

91. Can herpes be transmitted from the mother to the child?

Q. **How can an inactive herpes carrier prevent mother-to-child transmission of the virus, during and after pregnancy?**

A. If herpes is inactive, there is hardly any chance of transmission of herpes to child. Only if herpes genitalis is active at the time of delivery, then caesarean section is indicated. If you want to suppress an attack of herpes genitalis, then acyclovir 400 mg can be taken in the last month of pregnancy every 8 hourly. However, acyclovir has not been approved by the regulatory authorities for use during pregnancy and is labelled a category C drug (to be used only if the potential benefit outweighs the risk).

Herpes simplex virus (HSV) can be transmitted to the infant during the antenatal, intranatal or postnatal periods. In about 90% of cases, neonatal herpes is transmitted when an infant passes through an infected birth canal during delivery. Interestingly, 75%–90% of infants with neonatal HSV are born to asymptomatic mothers who have no history of HSV infection. There is a high risk of transmission if the mother has an active infection. There is also a small risk of transmission when the virus reactivates without causing any symptoms.

Five per cent of all cases of neonatal HSV infection result from transmission inside the uterus. There is a potential risk of HSV spreading through the blood to the placenta, and to the fetus. This can produce a number of other defects similar to other TORCH (Toxoplasmosis, Other infections, Rubella, Cytomegalovirus infection, and Herpes simplex) infections, e.g. microcephaly (small head), micro-ophthalmia (small eyes), calcifications in the brain and chorioretinitis (in the eye).

Women who are carriers of HSV infection should be screened for other sexually transmitted infections (STIs). Their partners should also be screened for STIs. A carrier can expect to have 2–4 symptomatic recurrences, especially during late pregnancy. Ten per cent of recurrences are asymptomatic. Care of babies born to carriers is important. Such newborns should be isolated and cultures should be taken from the eyes, pharynx (mouth) and skin for HSV infection at birth and after 24 hours. If positive, the newborn should be treated with antiviral therapy. There is no need to separate the baby from the mother. The mother should be instructed in proper hand-washing. Breastfeeding is allowed, unless there are lesions on the breast. Family members with oral herpetic lesions (herpes labialis) should not kiss the baby and should observe careful hand-washing methods.

92. Is abortion necessary if one is bitten by a dog?

Q. My sister is 2 months pregnant. Two weeks ago she was bitten by a dog and took an anti-rabies shot. On her next visit to the gynaecologist, it was suggested that she abort the baby because of the risk of neurological side-effects. My parents and her husband are very confused. Is there any such risk?

A. Your sister can take diploid cell vaccines. She doesn't need to abort.

People who are bitten by a dog and are not immunized should immediately wash all bite wounds and scratches with soap and water to decrease the chance of infection. Your sister should have had one injection of rabies immune globulin immediately after the bite, and the first dose of rabies vaccine. The immune globulin provides immediate protection from the virus. If your sister was not vaccinated previously she should be administered four additional doses of the rabies vaccine on the 3rd, 7th, 14th and 28th days after the bite. If she has been previously vaccinated, she needs to get only two doses of the vaccine – one right away and the other on the 3rd day. Rabies immune globulin is not required in previously vaccinated persons. The immune globulin and vaccine can be administered to pregnant women. One dose of tetanus toxoid should also be given.

93. Is a positive Toxoplasma IgM antibody harmful for the fetus?

Q. I am pregnant and I got my toxoplasmosis IgM and IgG titres tested in the 9th week of gestation. The results were negative for IgG but positive for IgM (48.7). This test was done using ELISA. What should I do now? Do I have to terminate my pregnancy? If not, is there any risk of passing the disease to the fetus? Will there be any abnormalities in the fetus? Will this infection affect my health? Do I need some medication for it? Can I get rid of this

infection forever? I don't know when I got infected with this. Do I need other confirmatory tests?

A. The IgM antibody indicates recent infection and IgG antibody past infection. Your IgM antibody titre is slightly higher than normal (positive). I advise you to get the test repeated immediately. Irrespective of whether this result is positive (low-positive) or high-positive or negative, I would advise you to repeat it a third time from the same laboratory (where the second testing is done) after two weeks.

At that time, the lab should test the sample drawn on the second occasion along with the sample drawn the third time to rule out any inter test error. Further management will depend upon these results. If the second and third samples are negative, you need not worry and have your ultrasound done regularly by an experienced sonologist. If the tests are positive (even if low-positive), I would advise you to have the pregnancy terminated. You can then (for documentation sake) get the aborted fetus sent for *Toxoplasma* isolation. However, that would just be a theoretical exercise. Chances of the baby getting infected are 15%, 30% and 60% (approximately) if acute infection in the mother occurs in the 1st, 2nd or 3rd trimester, respectively. One trimester is of 3 months.

It is no point going through cordocentesis (drawing of blood from the umbilical cord) and testing it for evidence of infection in the baby. It is a specialized procedure and very few obstetricians are competent enough to perform this test. Another test is amniotic fluid for polymerase chain reaction (PCR) of *Toxoplasma* or isolation of *Toxoplasma*. Very few research centres have these facilities. The chances of fetal wastage – abortion, death of the fetus and severe neurological complications (including hydrocephaly, microcephaly) – are highest when infection occurs in the 1st trimester and lowest or result in mild neurological problems when infection of the baby occurs in 3rd trimester. Even if tests show that the baby is not infected, he or she must be examined well and followed up to childhood to make sure there are no problems due to the congenital infection.

Drugs are available – spiramycin (which decreases the chance of congenital infection) and pyrimethamine–sulphadiazine combination. However, the last two drugs are not given before 14 weeks of pregnancy due to their harmful effects on the developing baby. In case you decide to abort the baby, before attempting the next pregnancy, you should be treated with these drugs and ensure that the IgG levels come down.

Infection confers immunity. Maternal chronic infection is not transmitted to the fetus. (*See also* page 18)

94. Can toxoplasmosis damage the fetus?

Q. Can *Toxoplasma* infection cause severe damage to the unborn baby? I am 36 years old and infected with it. I have had two pregnancies and lost both the babies. One had hydrocephaly and the next one was born alive but died after two weeks of delivery. My doctor says that the cause was toxoplasmosis. Please advise.

A. *Toxoplasma* infection during pregnancy can cause many problems in the fetus. Did you get treated for the infection after it was diagnosed? Once you are treated, you should only have antibodies in your blood and no active organism to cause trouble with future pregnancies. Please see an obstetrician to get another opinion on your unfavourable pregnancy outcomes.

95. Is it safe to treat malaria during pregnancy?

Q. I am 12–14 weeks pregnant and suspected to have malaria. Is it safe to consume quinolone drugs during pregnancy? Please mention the name of malaria drugs which are safe during pregnancy.

A. Malaria is a major risk to pregnancy. The high fever, chills and rigors that occur with malaria frequently cause premature birth, miscarriage and stillbirth. Experience with the recommended antimalarial drugs indicate that they are safe to take while pregnant; in fact, safer for you and your pregnancy than getting malaria. Usually, either chloroquine or mefloquine is prescribed for treatment.

Experience with chloroquine, and limited experience with mefloquine, indicates that they are safe to take during pregnancy, including the first trimester. Pregnant women should never take the following antimalarial drugs: atovaquone/proguanil, doxycycline or primaquine. These drugs are either not safe to take during pregnancy, or there is insufficient information currently to evaluate their safety.

Mefloquine has been recently used for chloroquine-resistant falciparum malaria, and accumulated reports point to its safety in pregnancy. Quinine is reserved for severe chloroquine-resistant malaria. Malformations were reported during the 1930s when quinine was used in large doses for inducing abortion. Malformations have not been reported when used in therapeutic doses for malaria. Quinine should be avoided if possible during pregnancy, but should not be withheld from severely ill women with malaria because of fetal concerns.

96. Is it safe to get a test for TB done during pregnancy?

Q. My employer wants me to get a TB test done. I am worried because I may be pregnant but it is still too early to tell. Is it safe to get a PPD test done when one is pregnant?

A. Tuberculin skin testing is safe and reliable for pregnant women. Purified protein derivative (PPD) does not cause malformations in the fetus. However, it is best to inform your employer regarding the pregnancy. The employer can discuss with the company doctor the need to get the test done during the pregnancy.

Routine testing of pregnant women is not necessary, unless you have conditions which suggest a high risk of progression from infection to disease. These conditions include:

- Symptoms suggestive of active TB disease
- HIV infection or behavioural risk factors for HIV infection, where the HIV status is unknown
- Recently arrived foreign-born people from areas where TB disease is endemic, e.g. Asia, Africa, Russia, Latin America, the Caribbean, etc.
- Medical conditions that have been reported to increase the risk of TB disease, such as diabetes mellitus, silicosis, prolonged corticosteroid therapy, other immunosuppressive therapy, haematological reticuloendothelial diseases (e.g. leukaemia and Hodgkin disease), carcinoma of the head, neck or lung, end-stage renal disease, intestinal bypass or gastrectomy, chronic malabsorption syndromes, or low body weight (10% or more below ideal weight)
- Close contact of someone with infectious laryngeal or TB lung disease.

97. What happens if a woman tests positive for hepatitis B during pregnancy?

Q. I am 28 years old and this is the 14th week of my first pregnancy. When we had the first blood test (I am O-negative), I was found to be positive for hepatitis B. When we did the same test last year, I was normal. Is this a big problem? What is the preferred diet for me?

A. In your case it is important to: (1) Confirm that the test is actually positive; (2) if it is positive, you should establish whether the disease is active or chronic, by blood tests for IgM anti-HBc, HBeAg, anti-HBe, and IgG anti-HBc. If you have IgM anti-HBc, and HBeAg, with the absence of anti-HBe and IgG anti-HBc, it shows that you have active disease and are highly infectious for your husband and the baby. About 10% of babies get infected if maternal active disease occurs in the first trimester and 80%–90% get infected if infection occurs in the third trimester. In chronic infection, infection of the baby occurs during delivery and later during breastfeeding. You should also be tested for hepatitis C, HIV and other sexually transmitted infections (STIs). After delivery a physician should follow you up regularly.

Your husband or partner also needs to be tested for HBsAg, and other STIs. If he tests negative for HBsAg, he should receive hepatitis B immunoglobulin and vaccine. He also needs to use condoms during vaginal intercourse.

The baby should receive hepatitis B immunoglobulin at birth as well as the vaccine. Untreated infected newborns can be carriers and 70%–90% will ultimately develop liver cancer. However, breastfeeding is not contraindicated, i.e. you can continue with it.

Needless to say, the doctors, nurses and paramedical staff should observe standard precautions during your blood testing and delivery.

98. How can the fetus be protected if the mother is HBsAg positive?

Q. What is the best option to treat a 5 months' pregnant patient who is HBsAg positive, to protect both the baby and the mother?

A. It is not very clear from your query whether there is an acute infection (active infection) or just a positive HBsAg. As HBsAg screening is routinely done nowadays, we detect it in people with no symptoms at all. If you have no obvious symptoms you could just be a carrier without having acute asymptomatic disease. To differentiate between the two (as the two have different prognoses): if you are found to be positive on routine testing, a liver function test and HBeAb and HBeAg are essential at this stage. (HBcAb and HBsAb are not required as they are unhelpful.)

If you have acute hepatic infection, you have to be under the care of a gastroenterologist/perinatal physician. Not much in the form of treatment can be given even if you have acute infection, but special care is required - general care and nutrition, as the prognosis of acute infection is worse in a pregnant than in a non-pregnant woman. So, you will require further care only if you have an acute infection but you need not bother if you are a carrier (only HBsAg positive and other reports normal, with no symptoms). The risk of transmission to the fetus is there and nothing much can be done at this stage to prevent it. Once the baby is born, an expert neonatologist will check the baby to exclude hepatitis B virus (HBV) positivity. Once the baby is negative for HBV, the baby will be given immunoglobulins and specific HBV vaccine which ensures 90% protection if used within hours/days of delivery. Those not covered by it are assumed to have had an intrauterine infection. The concern of passing the infection to the infant is genuine and you need to deliver in a good centre with expert neonatal care available round the clock or bring the baby to a special neonatal unit hours after delivery for testing and follow-up action.

99. Can CMV infection lead to repeated abortions?

Q. I am 30 years old and married for 6 years. I have yet not been blessed with a child, even though I have been able to conceive. The first time I conceived was 6 years ago but I aborted it in 45 days because of certain family problems. I was able to conceive only 4 years after that. But this pregnancy too did not last long and I suffered a missed abortion within 6 weeks. I tested positive for rubella antibodies and CMV (both IgG), but I did not take any medication. I am at present under treatment for infertility and under medication for CMV. I underwent an IUI last month and tested positive for pregnancy in 31 days after the LMP, but this pregnancy also did not last. In both the cases I underwent a D&C. I again tested positive for CMV. Is CMV the cause for both my missed abortions? I read on the internet that CMV cannot be treated. Does that mean that I will never have a child? Please help.

A. It is unlikely that the cytomegalovirus (CMV) infection is the cause of your 2 missed abortions at or less than 6 weeks of pregnancy. First-time infection with CMV (primary infection) during pregnancy has a 20%–50% chance of transmission to the fetus (baby), and of these infected fetuses, about 1%–2% have obvious disease at birth.

Women once infected with CMV, and who have latent infection, can have reactivation during pregnancy. Rates of reactivation are not known and differ from population to population. Prevention is by observing clean practices and avoiding being near people, especially children, who have colds. Usually one gets infected with CMV from nasopharyngeal secretions, infected urine and, of course, sexual intercourse. Infection is commonest among children aged 5 years or less. I guess you are not teaching in a nursery school or working in a creche. In such women (with reactivation during pregnancy), chances of transmission to the fetus is ~1%. So, the chances of your fetus getting infected next time you get pregnant are extremely low. However, you need to be properly monitored during your next pregnancy for reactivation of infection.

If pregnancy is proved, you need to undergo tests: usually ultrasound is done, as it is non-invasive, to look for signs of infection in the fetus. Cordocentesis (drawing blood from the umbilical cord when the baby is still in the uterus) is a highly specialized technique that can be done only by trained doctors. Blood so drawn can be tested for CMV. In case the baby is proven to be infected, it should be examined closely at birth and later to see if he/she develops signs of infection. If the baby's infection is not diagnosed before birth, this should be done immediately at birth.

In short, the CMV infection you have cannot result in missed abortion at 6 weeks. I would advise you to be tested for other causes – endocrinological, immunological and genetic causes. I suggest you put yourself under the care of an experienced obstetrician in your city. Next time you conceive, you should be registered under someone who is working in a major hospital where all test facilities are available.

100. I am HIV-positive but my pregnant wife is not. Can my child be infected?

Q. I have tested HIV positive. My wife is pregnant now (5 months) but she is negative. What do I do now? Please advise.

A. First get a confirmatory test (Western blot or repeat ELISA using different HIV antigens) for HIV done for yourself. If negative, stop worrying and forget about it. If positive, you need to be evaluated completely and treated. Your wife, you say, is HIV negative. The test should be repeated after 3 months and 6 months (if negative at 3 months). If she tests positive, she should be screened for other STIs, and her CD4 counts done. The CD4 counts will dictate the need for antiviral treatment, the number of drugs, and prognosis for the mother as well as the fetus. Toxoplasma, recurrent cytomegalovirus (CMV) and herpes simplex virus (HSV) infections, influenza, and pneumococcal infections are common in HIV-positive women. She should be vaccinated with hepatitis B, influenza and pneumococcal vaccines. Counselling of both the husband and the wife is very important.

Can you guess when you got infected? Was it during the pregnancy or before? If during the pregnancy, did you have sex with your wife during this time? If you did, then for the sake of your unborn child you must assume that your wife is infected but in the window period. She should therefore be put on antiretrovirals to prevent transmission to the baby. Consult your doctor for a suitable prescription. One drug that is used is nevirapine, one dose to the mother during labour and one to the child soon after delivery. If you can afford it, avoid breastfeeding the child. If you cannot afford artificial feeds, ensure that the child does not take anything else other than breast milk. Not even water, for 3–4 months. Lastly, consult your doctor regarding an elective caesarean section to minimize exposure to blood etc. during delivery. Please use a condom when you have sex with your wife.

If a woman tests positive for HIV and is ≤20 weeks pregnant, the option for medical termination of pregnancy should be offered. The HIV-positive pregnant woman is at a higher risk for preterm labour, fetal growth restriction and stillbirth.

101. Can a pregnant woman transmit HIV infection to her unborn child?

Q. I have heard that the chances of vertical transmission of AIDS is around 30%–40%, which means 60%–70% of babies won't have any HIV infection at all. Is this true?

A. Without treatment, there is a 60%–70% chance that the baby born to an HIV-positive mother will not have vertically transmitted HIV infection. However, the probability of HIV infection in the baby can be considerably reduced by treatment of the mother and child. Even one dose of an appropriate medicine, to the mother during labour and to the baby within 72 hours of birth, reduces the chance of infection considerably. This is available free of cost at many places as a part of the Government's programme to prevent parent-to-child transmission of HIV. More rigorous regimens reduce the total probability to 1%–2%. Breastfeeding must be avoided to cut down the chance of infection but this can obviously only be done if the mother can afford adequate and safe alternate feeds for the baby.

102. How dangerous is chicken pox during pregnancy?

Q. My wife is 22 weeks pregnant and is suffering from chicken pox. How serious is it for the mother and the child? She is taking Crocin for fever and amoxycillin as advised. This has helped her a lot. Please advise whether there will be any complications for the child or mother.

A. Chicken pox can lead to pneumonitis (lung infection with the virus) in the pregnant woman and can be rather serious. However, the disease seems to be under control. Infection of the mother in the first 20 weeks of pregnancy can cause congenital malformations of the baby such as skin lesions, bony leg defects, hydronephrosis (enlargement of the kidneys), infection of the eyes (chorioretinitis) and the brain can also get affected (cortical atrophy); these occur in about 2% of cases (maximum between 13 and 20 weeks of pregnancy). Your wife has just crossed that period. The incubation period of this virus is short – less than 2 weeks; so hopefully she has caught the infection soon after 20 weeks or at the end of 20 weeks.

Infection in the latter half of pregnancy is associated with congenital varicella (chicken pox) lesions and occasionally zoster (a variant of chicken pox) develops several months later. Fetal exposure just before or after delivery (within 5 days), before maternal protective antibodies form and cross the placenta into the baby, can be a serious threat to the newborn. In such cases, varicella zoster immunoglobulin (VZIG) is administered to the newborn. Despite this, roughly 15% of newborns develop serious life-threatening infection.

Most women are already immune from prior infection or immunization in childhood. If not immune, the woman should be vaccinated with VZIG after delivery, within 96 hours of exposure. The vaccine should not be administered to pregnant women.

Except for the bony leg defect and the hydronephrosis (kidney problem), which can be detected by ultrasound (done by an expert), it is not possible to diagnose unequivocally any of the other possible conditions that could affect the baby before birth. Have a good paediatrician available at the time of delivery, so that he or she examines the baby thoroughly and conducts the necessary tests.

103. Is there a risk of re-infection after one episode of shingles during pregnancy?

Q. My wife is 22 weeks pregnant. She had a mild case of shingles at 17 weeks. Blood tests show that she is not immune to varicella, but has had chicken pox as a child. We know there are chances of complications in the first trimester and close to delivery. She is a schoolteacher and is due in March. Chicken pox is common at that time of year, especially with about 500 schoolchildren. We are very concerned. She was planning to work until her delivery. Should she stop working now that she has had shingles and has no immunity to varicella?

A. Since she has had this episode now, there is practically no risk of developing a recurrence/re-infection.

It is surprising that your wife had chicken pox in childhood and has tested not immune for varicella. The test needs to be repeated. Shingles (herpes zoster) and chicken pox are caused by the same virus. The chicken pox virus may remain dormant in the nerve roots and can be reactivated after many years to cause shingles. Maternal zoster is more common in older and immunocompromised women. Therefore, your wife needs to have other diseases that lead to suppressed immunity ruled out. There is no evidence that zoster is more serious in pregnant women. There is little evidence of shingles (zoster) causing congenital malformations.

The diagnosis of 'mild shingles' also needs to be reviewed. You also need to be tested for varicella immunity if you have not suffered from it earlier. If you are not immune, you need to receive varicella zoster immune globulin (VZIG) (if it is within 96 hours of exposure), and also the vaccine. If both of you have children who are not immune to varicella, they also need to be vaccinated.

104. What is the treatment for scabies during pregnancy?

Q. What is the treatment of scabies during pregnancy?

A. Application of sulphur (10%) ointment locally all over the body, below the neck, daily at night for 3 days and similarly, application of crotamiton ointment for 3 days are safe in pregnancy. To control itching, application of crotamiton ointment may be continued for 2 weeks or so.

Application of 1%–10% gamma benzene hexachloride or a 12.5%–25% suspension of benzyl benzoate is very effective. These agents should be applied from neck downwards after a bath. The treatment should be repeated after 3 days.

Good personal hygiene is important. Secondary skin infection, if present, should be treated with systemic antibiotics (erythromycin or penicillin). Examination and treatment of family members and close contacts is important, as well as pets (though the species that infects animals rarely infects man).

105. If a pregnant woman gets chikungunya, will it harm the fetus?

Q. If a pregnant woman, in her second trimester, suffers from chikungunya, will this harm the fetus? If yes, what are the effects?

A. If a mother gets chikungunya virus infection between 3–4.5 months into pregnancy; mother-to-fetus infection can occur. Before and after that period in pregnancy, infection has not been reported. However, there is a 48% risk of infection at birth if the virus is still present in the mother's blood.

Such an infection may cause miscarriages, but any increase in cases of birth defects has not been seen. Fever, in general, can trigger uterine contractions, miscarriage or cause fetal death.

106. Are raised liver enzymes common during pregnancy?

Q. My wife is 34 weeks pregnant. Recently, she did some blood tests. The results are: haemoglobin (Hb): 10.8; RBC: 4.63; bilirubin: 1.5; SGPT: 268 and SGOT: 260. I know they are very high. Is this common during pregnancy? What should we do?

A. No single liver function can quantify or define liver disease and a panel of laboratory tests profiling discrete aspects of liver functions (called liver function tests) are required. An injury to the liver cells (necrosis) is measured by determining aspartate aminotransferase (AST) and alanine aminotransferase (ALT) levels, while the synthetic function of liver is quantified by determining albumin level and prothrombin time. This may be affected in cirrhosis or severe hepatic disease. Measurement of bilirubin, alkaline phosphatase and gamma glutamyl transferase (GGT) define obstructive liver disease (cholestasis and biliary obstruction). In normal pregnancy, alkaline phosphatase levels may increase up to 4 times, secondary to placental alkaline phosphatase levels.

Elevation of ALT during pregnancy can be a result of viral hepatitis which can be easily diagnosed using serological tests. Other possible causes of mild or moderate elevation of ALT are drug-induced hepatotoxicity, hyperemesis gravidarum, cholelithiasis, HELLP (haemolysis, elevated liver enzymes and low platelet count) syndrome or acute fatty liver of pregnancy. If viral hepatitis is ruled out, the elevated enzymes have to be viewed in the clinical context of the patient and appropriate investigations should be done.

Metabolic disorders

107. Can I conceive if I am MTHR-positive?

Q. I am 42 years old. I have been considering having another child for 2 years now. I had some blood tests done and tested positive for MTHR. I am taking folic acid and vitamins B6 and B12. Can I still go ahead with the baby? Is it much harder at this age to conceive, and any suggestions on when to conceive? I would appreciate your input. I had a miscarriage 2 years ago.

A. MTHR stands for methylene tetrahydrofolate reductase, an enzyme which is present in the cells of our body to metabolize and get rid of homocysteine. High homocysteine levels are a risk factor for blood clots in the veins (deep vein thrombosis, pulmonary embolism) or arteries (heart attack, stroke, arteriosclerosis). Some individuals have a variant of this enzyme, which is called thermolabile MTHR or C677T/MTHR, caused by a single mutation of the MTHR gene. This variant does not metabolize homocysteine as well as the normal MTHR enzyme, and blood homocysteine levels in individuals with this variant enzyme may therefore be slightly higher than in individuals with the normal enzyme.

There are three likely possibilities—either one does not have the MTHR mutation, or one is heterozygous (1 variant gene), or homozygous (2 variant genes). It is only the homozygous mutation that is associated with elevated homocysteine levels. Nearly half the population may be MTHR heterozygous so it is nothing abnormal and does not cause elevation of homocysteine levels. The fasting homocysteine level should be measured and, if normal, there is no need for vitamin B or folate therapy - even if you have the homozygous MTHR mutation.

Individuals with MTHR mutation who have normal homocysteine levels are not at increased risk for clots. Raised homocysteine levels may also be due to vitamin B and folate deficiency and renal failure. Often we do not know why the levels are raised.

Levels can be lowered by taking a multivitamin with a high content of folic acid, vitamin B6 (pyridoxine) and vitamin B12 (cobalamine). Often, folate treatment alone lowers homocysteine levels sufficiently. Approximately two months after starting vitamins, the homocysteine level should be checked again to make sure it has returned to normal.

Coming to the age-related question, studies have demonstrated that almost 50% of women over the age of 40 experience infertility as fertility in women decreases with advancing age. This age-associated decline in fertility (and increase in miscarriages) is largely due to abnormalities in the egg itself, less frequent ovulation or to problems such as endometriosis, in which tissue similar to that lining the uterus gets attached to the ovaries or fallopian tubes and interferes with conception.

The rate of miscarriage in older women is significantly greater than that in younger women. The increased incidence of chromosomal abnormalities contributes to this age-related risk of miscarriage. Women over the age of 40 have an approximately one-in-three chance of having a miscarriage in any given pregnancy. In addition, 1 in 60 live births is genetically abnormal. High rates of abnormal chromosome distribution are a major factor that can explain the lower rate of successful pregnancies in older women. There is also a greater chance of bearing twins. Women over 35 also have an increased risk of placental problems. The most common placental problem is placenta praevia, in which the placenta covers (partially or completely) the opening of the cervix. Fetal distress and a prolonged second stage of labour are more common in older mothers. There is also an increased risk of having a baby who is of low birth weight or premature, and increased risk of ectopic pregnancy (in which the fertilized egg is implanted outside the uterus, usually in the fallopian tube).

There are some special considerations for the older woman trying to conceive. These would include general health issues, since women over 40 are more likely to have medical problems, e.g. diabetes, hypertension, heart disease – which can complicate a pregnancy. Therefore, an older woman contemplating a pregnancy should undergo a thorough medical evaluation, including a mammogram. Due to the increased incidence of genetic abnormalities in infants born to women above the age of 40, prenatal chorionic villus sampling or amniocentesis may be required.

I have listed out most of the problems that you are likely to face. At the same time, please understand that even though older women face some special risks, many of these risks can be managed effectively with good prenatal care. It is important to keep in mind that the increased risk, even for the oldest women, is modest. Today, most women in their late 30s and 40s who are planning a pregnancy can look forward to having a normal pregnancy and a healthy baby.

The cause for the previous miscarriage also needs to be investigated. You need to discuss all these issues with your obstetrician and plan your pregnancy. All the best! (*See also* page 142)

108. Should high uric acid levels be treated?

Q. I have a high level of uric acid (9.2 mg/dl) and I am taking 2 tablets of Zyloric daily. This is my 4th week of pregnancy. Would you advise me to continue with this pregnancy or terminate it fearing that it could lead to complications for the baby? I had an abortion at 5 weeks due to agenesis of the corpus callosum. I have a son who is as normal as a child of 9 years can be. I had a medical termination of pregnancy 5 years ago.

A. A high uric acid does not require any treatment unless it has caused acute gouty attacks. By itself high uric acid is simply indicative of a poor lifestyle (lack of exercise and excess calories in a diet that is low in fibre, leafy vegetables and fruits). I strongly recommend that you see a good general physician who would advise you on these problems. To the best of my knowledge, a young woman should not take Zyloric unless advised by an expert in metabolic diseases.

Allopurinol (Zyloric) is relatively contraindicated during pregnancy. It is used for both primary (due to gout) and secondary hyperuricaemia (seen in haematological disorders and with antineoplastic therapy). Allopurinol is associated with facial clefts and minor skeletal abnormalities in mice; its effects on the human fetus are unknown. It can be used during breastfeeding. In rare cases such as this, it is best to consult the medical specialist. In fact, women with these disorders should first consult their doctor regarding treatment before planning a pregnancy.

109. How can one manage gestational diabetes?

Q. I am 28 years old and in the 34th week of my second pregnancy. I am

expecting twins. My doctor advised a GTT. The readings of my test are: FBS 5.4 mmol/L (mg/dl), 1st hour 9.7 mmol/L, 2nd hour 8.5 mmol/L. Do I have diabetes as per the above results? Is there a chance of having it in future? My father was diabetic. What is the normal range of glucose in the blood during pregnancy?

A. You have what is called gestational diabetes. Get your HbA1c (glycosylated haemoglobin) done – it should be <7%. Also try to keep your 2-hour post-meal blood glucose around 120–130 mg%.

Your blood sugar is expected to come down to the normal range after delivery, but you are under greater risk for development of diabetes. Therefore, after delivery, regular exercise, maintaining a normal body weight, and lifestyle modifications for a stress-free life are important to prevent diabetes.

The cut-off values for plasma glucose (in mg/dl) for diagnosing impaired glucose tolerance or gestational diabetes by the 100 g oral glucose tolerance test (GTT) are as follows:

Time of measurement	Plasma glucose level	
	National Diabetes Data Group, USA (1979) (in mg/dl)	Carpenter and Coustan (1982) (in mg/dl)
Fasting	105	95
1 hour	190	180
2 hours	165	155
3 hours	145	140

Gestational diabetes is diagnosed when any two values are met or exceeded.

The World Health Organization (WHO) recommends the 75 g oral GTT with 2-hour values. The cut-offs for diagnosing impaired glucose tolerance are: Fasting ≤7.8 mmol/L; 2-hour value ≥8 mmol/L and ≤11 mmol/L. Diabetes mellitus is diagnosed if the fasting glucose is >7.8 mmol/L and/or 2-hour glucose is >11 mmol/L. As these values are based on the non-pregnant population, the European group has suggested higher cut-offs: 1-hour glucose ≥10.5 mmol/L and 2-hour glucose ≥9 mmol/L and ≤11 mmol/L.

The goals for self-monitored capillary blood glucose during pregnancy in diabetic women are: fasting: 60–90 mg/dl (3.3–5.0 mmol), pre-meal: 60–105 mg/dl (3.3–5.8 mmol), 1-hour postprandial: 100–120 mg/dl (5.5–6.7 mmol), and 2 hours after meals: 60–120 mg/dl (3.3–6.7 mmol).

Patients with gestational diabetes should undergo a 75 g oral GTT at 6 and 12 weeks after delivery. If the tests are normal, the test should be repeated at a minimum of 3-year intervals for early detection of type 2 diabetes mellitus. Women with gestational diabetes have a 50% likelihood of developing overt diabetes within 20 years of delivery. If fasting hyperglycaemia develops during pregnancy, it is more likely to persist after delivery.

110. What are the precautions to be taken in case of gestational diabetes?

Q. My wife was diagnosed with gestational diabetes in her 30th week of pregnancy. She is on a strict diabetic diet, goes for a one-hour walk every day and takes 14 units of insulin twice daily. Her doctor has told her to maintain post-meal 1-hour sugar levels up to 140 mg/dl. Her readings generally come in the 135–145 mg/dl range. I read somewhere that post-meal 1-hour sugar levels for pregnant women should be less than 120–130 mg/dl. Can you clarify what level should she maintain?

A. Strict control of blood sugar levels is the key to a good outcome for both the mother and her baby. Family support is equally important.

During a healthy pregnancy, the average fasting blood sugar levels show a remarkably low value of 74±2.7 (standard deviation) mg/dl. On the other hand, the peak postprandial or post-meal blood sugar values rarely exceed 120 mg/dl. This is known to reduce the rate of macrosomia or unusually large babies. For example, when the 2-hour post-meal glucose levels are maintained at less than 120 mg/dl, approximately 20% of fetuses have macrosomia. Conversely, if the postprandial levels are up to 160 mg/dl, the macrosomia rate rises to 35%.

The current recommendations are:

- Fasting whole blood glucose level should be less than 95 mg/dl (5.3 mmol/L)
- Two-hour postprandial whole blood glucose level should be less than 120 mg/dl (6.7 mmol/L)

The basic management of your wife's condition can be done through dietary control, regular home glucose monitoring and insulin therapy.

Most patients with gestational diabetes mellitus (GDM) diagnosed in the third trimester, such as your wife, can maintain 1-hour postprandial blood glucose levels less than 130 mg/dl via diet manipulation (for example, she should have small, more frequent and non-glycaemic [without sugar] meals and should exercise).

Home glucose monitoring is essential to help your wife choose the type and timing of meals. For the first 1–2 weeks, she should perform capillary glucose checks first thing after waking up (fasting) and 1 hour after each major meal. Mid-morning, mid-afternoon and bedtime snacks are essential to blunt or lessen the rise in glucose levels after meals.

Once her post-meal glucose levels are controlled with diet, the occurrence of abnormal fasting levels is exceedingly rare and the morning checks can be discontinued. Fasting checks are to be restarted if the postprandial glucose level is abnormal.

Recent research shows that the earlier insulin therapy is started, the better the outcome. Treatment with insulin reduces the chances of having a very large and fat baby.

Insulin treatment is based on individual glucose profiles. When more than 20% of the post-meal blood sugar values are above 130 mg/dl, administering rapid-acting insulin injections (4–8 units to start with) before meals is usually successful in controlling the increase in glucose levels. If more than 10 units of rapid-acting insulin are needed before the noon meal, adding 6–12 units dose of neutral protamine hagedorn (NPH) insulin before breakfast helps achieve smoother control. When more than 10% of the fasting glucose levels are above 95 mg/dl, a starting dose of 6–8 units of NPH insulin can be used at bedtime. The doses are increased once or twice weekly as necessary to keep the glucose levels in check.

Care of the pregnant diabetic woman is a team effort between the endocrinologist, obstetrician, ultrasonologist and neonatologist. Your wife should register for delivery in a hospital with a good neonatal intensive care unit.

111. How can sugar levels be maintained in gestational diabetes?

Q. I am a 27-year-old woman and am 9 months pregnant. I have been diagnosed as having gestational diabetes. I am on human insulin Mixtard

morning 28 and night 10 units. My weight is 65 kg. Every week I undergo a blood test. Last week my PPBS was 160. Would I deliver normally or by caesarean section? Ultrasound scan and everything else is normal, the doctor says. What precautions do I have to take to avoid C-section?

A. The chances of a C-section are certainly more if you have any medical problem, and that includes diabetes, but that does not mean you will definitely have a C-section.

Precautions include: maintaining good control by walking regularly, eating a diet in which fats are not in excess, doing home blood glucose monitoring (just lab tests are usually not enough). However, most of these would have been more useful if done earlier on: now that you are already 9 months pregnant, and the delivery is around the corner, stay active (as much walking as you can manage) and stay calm.

112. What should be the diet during pregnancy if one is a diabetic?

Q. What should be done when a woman becomes diabetic during the 7th month of pregnancy? What diet and which medicines should she follow?

A. A normal diet without direct sugar is recommended. Sweets, confectionery, chocolates, etc. should be avoided. Small, frequent meals are desirable.

113. What care should a diabetic take during pregnancy?

Q. I am 29 years old and have type 1 diabetes for the past 12 years. My wife aged 29 years is also a type 1 diabetic since 11 years of age. Recently, her blood sugar level became very high but her urine test was normal with no infection. We tested for pregnancy and it was positive. I am very worried about her glucose level, it is more than 300 mg/dl. Is it dangerous for the baby and the mother? What is the possibility of the baby having diabetes? Is there a chance of abnormality in the baby due to the high blood sugar level? What tests should we do to ensure/evaluate the health condition of both the baby and the mother?

A. If the father has type 1 diabetes, the risk is about 1 in 10 (10%) that his child will develop type 1 diabetes and if the mother (as she is 29) has type 1 diabetes, the risk is much lower, a little more than 10%.

Pregnant women with diabetes who have high blood glucose levels before or during pregnancy are more likely to have complications, including miscarriage, stillbirth, a large baby that requires a caesarean delivery, or worsening of existing kidney function or retinopathy. Birth defects are more common in women with raised blood glucose levels before and during the early weeks of pregnancy. There is no particular birth defect caused by maternal diabetes, though most defects occur by the 7th week of pregnancy. In earlier studies, the frequency of birth defects was approximately 8%–13% among diabetic women, compared with 2%–4% in the non-diabetic population. However, more recent studies have demonstrated that tight control of blood glucose before becoming pregnant greatly reduces the risk of birth defects to a level similar to women who do not have diabetes. First or second trimester screening for birth defects such as spina bifida and Down syndrome is recommended (for all women, not just those with diabetes). Women with diabetes are not at increased risk for having a baby with a chromosomal abnormality, such as Down syndrome, but they are at increased risk for having a baby with a neural tube defect (e.g. spina bifida).

These tests are used for screening (as opposed to diagnosis), and cannot determine with certainty if a baby has these problems. If the test is abnormal, an ultrasound examination and/or amniocentesis may be performed to determine if the abnormality is actually present. The infant of the diabetic mother is at risk for several problems in the newborn period, such as low blood glucose levels (less than 30 mg/dl [1.7 mmol/L]), jaundice, too many red blood cells (polycythaemia), low calcium level and heart problems. These problems are more common when the mother's blood glucose levels have been raised during the pregnancy. Most of these problems resolve within a few hours or days of delivery. Infants of diabetic mothers are often evaluated in a special care nursery for these potential problems.

Most women with good control of diabetes can expect an excellent outcome of pregnancy as a result of improvements in blood glucose control; this requires frequent daily glucose testing and insulin adjustment. We use 4 injections (3 short- or rapid-acting and one long-acting) a day, which can improve control and reduce the risk to the mother and the baby. Target blood glucose levels during pregnancy are as follows: HbA1c level: 6 mmol/L; Fasting blood glucose: 60–90 mg/dl (3.3–5 mmol/L); before meals: less than 100 mg/dl (5.5 mmol/L); one hour after meals: less than 130–140 mg/dl (7.2–7.7 mmol/L); two hours after meals: less than 120 mg/dl (6.7 mmol/L).

Postpartum (after delivery) care for a woman with diabetes is similar to that for a woman without diabetes. However, insulin requirements are highly variable in the immediate postpartum period; some women require little or no insulin. Insulin requirements usually return to near pre-pregnancy levels within 48 hours.

Breastfeeding is strongly encouraged, and benefits both the infant and the mother. Insulin requirements may be lower while breastfeeding, and frequent blood glucose monitoring is important to prevent severe hypoglycaemia. Approximately 400 additional calories are required each day while breastfeeding. Breastfeeding for longer than 3 months can aid in maternal weight loss and provides significant short- and long-term benefits to the infant.

A woman and her obstetrician may decide to schedule the date of her delivery (either an induction of labour or caesarean section), especially if there are risk factors, such as poor blood glucose levels, nephropathy, worsening retinopathy, hypertension or pre-eclampsia, or limited or excessive fetal growth. Waiting for labour to start on its own is reasonable if the blood glucose levels are well controlled and the mother and fetus are without problems. However, extending the pregnancy beyond 40–41 weeks of gestation is generally not recommended.

114. Can natural remedies help to control diabetes during pregnancy?

Q. I am 31 years old and 25 weeks pregnant. I was diagnosed with gestational diabetes 3 weeks back, and was put on insulin. For the past 3 days I have been trying a natural remedy in addition to my insulin dose. I have been drinking the juice of 1–2 small bitter gourds (*karela*) mixed with 2 gooseberries (*amla*) and have achieved significant control of my sugar levels. Is this mixture harmful, if consumed in a small quantity once a day, in the last trimester?

A. Therapeutic diet plays an important role in the treatment of diabetes. Nothing helps more than a diet, custom-made by a dietician. The general principle is to control body fat, which reduces the sensitivity to insulin and keeps a check on the blood sugar level.

A diabetic diet must include a balance of high proteins, low fat and complex carbohydrates (whole grain cereals, whole wheat flour, vegetables) which are digested more slowly and therefore do not cause a rapid rise in blood sugar.

The most important diet consideration is the total amount of calories ingested. For an average diabetic, about 60% of calories are derived from carbohydrates, 15%–20% from fats, and 15%–20% from proteins.

There are also several known home remedies to help keep the blood sugar levels in control.

Bitter gourd contains plant insulin and 2 ounces should be taken raw twice daily on an empty stomach. It is found to be very effective for diabetes. Or it can be cooked as a vegetable and eaten. Bitter gourd can also be powderd and crushed after drying. Take bitter gourd powder 1 teaspoon daily, on an empty stomach.

In the last trimester, please monitor your blood glucose level regularly and check with your physician to ensure that this does not contradict any medication that he might give you. The blood sugar levels should not fall below the normal levels.

Medications

115. Are iron supplements necessary during pregnancy?

Q. Why has the doctor prescribed Orofer XT of Emcure company to my wife? It is a ferrous ascorbate tablet, i.e. 100 mg elemental iron per tablet, whereas I have read that the RDA of iron during pregnancy is just 30 mg per day.

A. The Indian recommended daily allowance (RDA) for iron is 38 mg/ day during pregnancy and 30 mg/day during lactation (breastfeeding). During pregnancy there is a large requirement for iron, especially during the second half of pregnancy. This amount is not available from body stores in most women, and the maternal red blood cell volume and haemoglobin will fall if iron supplements are not given or are inadequate. The amount of iron absorbed from the diet together with that mobilized from the body stores is insufficient to meet the demands of pregnancy. The fetus will have adequate haemoglobin, because the placenta gets sufficient iron from the mother, even in anaemic women (the fetus is like a parasite). However, the baby's iron stores will be deficient after birth.

Only 5%–10% of ingested iron is absorbed. Iron absorption from the usual Indian diet is less than 5% because of the diet, which is rich in phytates (these inhibit iron absorption). A minimum of 6 mg of elemental iron must be absorbed daily to maintain the iron balance during pregnancy. Even if iron absorption is 10% of that ingested, one needs to have a diet containing 60 mg of iron. This level is impossible to achieve even with the best of diets. The usual diet cannot meet the increased requirement during pregnancy. Hence, iron supplementation during pregnancy is a must. In fact, it is mandatory for every pregnant woman to take 100 tablets of iron and folic acid during the second half of the pregnancy to prevent anaemia, as is being ensured by the Reproductive and Child Health Programme of the Government of India. Approximately 50% of all pregnant Indian women are anaemic and anaemia ranks first among the indirect causes of maternal death and disability in Indian women. Therefore, in a healthy woman with a singleton pregnancy, eating a nutritious balanced diet, probably an iron tablet containing 60 mg of elemental iron will be sufficient, provided she is regular, starts by the 16th week of pregnancy and has no malabsorption. Otherwise, a tablet containing 100 mg of elemental iron is required daily. If the woman is already anaemic, or has twins, she will require more than this.

116. Is it harmful to use aspirin during pregnancy?

Q. I am a 24-year-old married woman. I am 5 feet, 4 inches tall and weigh 54 kg. I had an abortion last year in the 9th month of my pregnancy. The doctor suspected it to be an accidental haemorrhage and later on there was some problem in the flow of blood in my body. I was operated and a 2 kg stillborn male fetus was delivered. It happened all of a sudden. Without any prior feeling of unease, I started bleeding profusely and was taken to the hospital immediately, where I was in labour for 6–7 hours. I was then operated upon and given 9 units of blood and fresh frozen plasma (FFP). It is a year since the incident. I want to plan for a baby again. I was suggested by a doctor to go for an antiphospholipid screen test. It was positive, and lupus antibodies (LA) confirmed. A thyroid stimulation test was done and the result was 1.63 uIU/ml, which is normal. My haemoglobin is 12 g/dl. My doctor suggested trying for a child by the natural method and I have started taking folic acid tablets as per her advice. However, she told me that from the time I conceive, I would be given a small amount of aspirin tablet every day till the 9th month of my pregnancy. I have read that aspirin is harmful during pregnancy. Please advise. I have no family history of any disease and I never had a miscarriage before.

A. Aspirin is given in small doses (not the dose used for fever or relieving pain) during pregnancy for certain definite indications, and it is beneficial. One of the indications is being positive for LA. I trust the confirmatory test was done. No doctor minds answering questions, especially when they are from patients like you who have gone through a rough time. Have trust in your obstetrician, and the Almighty. An important point to remember is that you should be under the care of an experienced obstetrician and be registered for delivery in a tertiary care hospital with all blood component facilities and a neonatal ICU.

Currently, the most effective treatment for women who test positive for LA, with previous bad obstetric outcome is low-dose aspirin (60–80 mg per day) along with low dose unfractionated heparin or low molecular weight heparin (e.g. enoxaprin). Aspirin in low doses has no adverse effect on the baby, though it is associated with a slight risk of bleeding from the small vessels during surgical procedures on the mother.

117. Is it harmful to use vitamin A cream during pregnancy?

Q. For the first trimester I used an under-eye cream. Later it was found that the cream had retinol acetate in it. A cosmetologist said that it is not harmful during pregnancy. Is retinol acetate different from Retin A? Is it safe to use it? I have stopped using it since then.

A. There are two forms of vitamin A in nature: *carotenoids*, especially beta-carotene, which is found in fruits and vegetables and has never been shown to cause birth defects, and *retinol* which is preformed vitamin A. Intake of vitamin A in doses higher than the RDA (recommended dietary allowance) during pregnancy should be avoided. Retrospective studies have shown that high doses of retinol (more than 10, 000 IU/day) are teratogenic (harmful to the unborn baby). The RDA (for Indian women) for vitamin A during pregnancy is the same as that before pregnancy and is 600 mcg/day of retinol. During lactation the RDA increases to 950 mcg/day.

Some creams and lotions used for dermatological (skin) conditions display the biological activity of vitamin A e.g. Retinol acctate in a cream is safe in pregnancy. Tretinoin is the active ingredient in Retin A, and is highly effective for cystic acne. It is highly teratogenic if used in the first trimester of pregnancy. A pregnancy test before starting treatment with this is mandatory.

Likewise, etretinate, which is used for the treatment of psoriasis, is teratogenic. It is suggested that women wait for at least 2 years after discontinuing treatment before conceiving. If possible, women who have not completed their family should not use this drug.

118. Why are Duvadilan and Susten taken during pregnancy?

Q. What is the purpose of consuming Duvadilan retard and Susten 200 during pregnancy? Is there any problem if I discontinue Susten 200 before completion of the course? I had muscular cramps and severe back pain from the very early stage of pregnancy. Also, I have noted blood stains in white discharge twice.

A. Duvadilan retard is the brand name of a medicine called isoxsuprine. It is a smooth muscle relaxant (it acts on arteries, muscles of the uterus, etc.) and was used to prevent premature labour. It is given towards the end of pregnancy if premature delivery is likely. Due to the entry of safer and more effective medicines, its use is no more in vogue in the US, UK, Australia, etc. It has no proven role in early pregnancy.

Susten is the brand name of a hormone called progesterone. It is to be given only when there is proven, documented deficiency of progesterone. In the past it was given as hormonal support during pregnancy. However, its use has become highly controversial since many experts now advise that it should not be used in pregnancy at all.

In Hungary, where 30% of all pregnant women were given progesterone, increased risk of developing hypospadias (urinary tube defect in male babies) and tetralogy of Fallot (serious defect in the development of the heart in the fetus) were reported. It can also cause masculinization of a female fetus (i.e. growth of facial hair etc.).

In conclusion, unless there is proven deficiency of progesterone, Susten should not be administered. Please consult your obstetrician again.

119. Is it safe to take Life, Folvite and Seroflo during pregnancy?

Q. I am 27 years old. After years of treatment, finally I conceived. Now I am 6 weeks pregnant. Cardiac activity is present and everything seems to be normal. My doctor has given me Life 5000 weekly and Folvite. Is it safe to take this injection weekly till the 16th week? I also have asthma and have been using Seroflo 125 inhaler, which contains steroids. Will this affect my baby?

A. You are still not 27 years old; hence I don't know why you underwent treatment for years. In any case Life is the brand name of a medicine called human chorionic gonadotrophin (hCG) that is given in certain selected cases up to 16 weeks of pregnancy. There will be no adverse effect.

Very small amounts of medicines are absorbed when taken through the inhalation route. Hence there is nothing to worry about taking Seroflo.

Shortage of folic acid can have very serious repercussions on the baby and Folvite containing folic acid is definitely recommended.

120. Can I take an enema during pregnancy?

Q. I am 4 months pregnant. I have the habit of straining after stools for complete evacuation. I felt this might cause a problem later in my pregnancy due to excess pressure on the abdomen. I bought an enema set and am using plain warm water for enema. I use it once in 3–4 days. Will this have any adverse effects on my colon? Will it cause any bad changes in the colonic environment? Will it make me prone to infections?

A. As you may be aware, most women tend to get constipated during pregnancy, which may worsen as the pregnancy advances. A soap and water enema is helpful and does no harm to the colon. However, there are mild laxatives that can be inserted in the back passage to facilitate bowel movement and, in my opinion, are better and easier alternatives. I suggest you consult your doctor for a laxative suppository suitable for you, as you may find it difficult to self-administer enemas as your pregnancy advances.

It is important to rule out other causes of constipation in this case as it is a 'habit', as you say, probably antedating pregnancy. Common causes include haemorrhoids (piles) and fissures in the anus. Other causes which are overlooked are various medicines leading to constipation, e.g. opiates, antidepressants, and some antacids containing calcium and aluminium. Other causes to be excluded are hypothyroidism and diabetes, and some inflammatory states of the bowel.

In order to prevent constipation and decrease the problem, do the following:

- Increase the fibre content of your diet by eating fruits and vegetables, bran cereal, whole wheat bread or *atta* and a high fibre diet (eating whole *dals* instead of skin-removed *dals*).
- Citrus fruits are especially good.

- Seedless dates, figs and prunes are good.
- A stool softener, such as dioctyl sodium sulphosuccinate, may be taken daily orally.
- Drink lots of fluids.
- One important point is bowel training. Make it a point to visit the toilet at a specified time each day - usually after 15–60 minutes of a large breakfast, since this is usually the time of maximal spontaneous propulsive motility of the bowel.
- Some exercise such as walking for 30 minutes twice a day, and being free of anxieties also help in relieving constipation.
- Some people suffer from constipation when taking iron supplements. The iron preparation and dosage can be changed after consulting the obstetrician.
- Bulk-forming laxatives such as *isabgol*, hyperosmotic laxatives such as sorbitol and lactulose are safe. Milk of Magnesia, a saline laxative, can also be used.

It is best to avoid self-administered enemas during pregnancy. It is important not to be constipated near term (delivery time), as impacted stools can not only cause lot of discomfort but can also hamper delivery of the baby.

121. What are the harmful effects of Cepodem if taken during pregnancy?

Q. My wife is 9 weeks pregnant. In the 5th week she had severe cough. The doctor gave her Honitus ayurvedic cough syrup but she did not get any relief. The doctor then gave her Cepodem-200 (cefpodoxime 200) for five days. Even then she didn't get relief, so she was given the antibiotic Doxinate (doxylamine + pyridoxine) for 5 days. After taking this she became fine and the medicine was stopped. I later found that Cepodem is not allowed in pregnancy. My wife has already taken it for five days during the 6th week of pregnancy. My wife's blood group is AB negative and this is her second pregnancy. After her first delivery the doctor gave her the injection required for a negative blood group mother. My first child was A+. I don't know the name of the injection. I am very scared about the coming child. What will be the impact of this medicine on him/her? Will the child be disabled? Should we go for an abortion? My wife is fine though.

A. Cefpodoxime is a kind of penicillin. Animal studies have shown that it does not cause any harm to the unborn baby. However, due to ethical reasons similar tests cannot be done in humans and therefore its safety in human pregnancy has not been established. This does not mean that it is unsafe. There is absolutely no reason to terminate the pregnancy. Just for the sake of abundant precaution and peace of mind, the development of the baby should be followed through serial ultrasound examinations.

Cefpodoxime is a reserve medicine – not first-line treatment for respiratory infections. It is generally prescribed for either recurrent or chronic respiratory tract infections that do not respond to other antibiotics. Most acute respiratory tract infections in India are due to viruses for which no medicine works except time.

Incidentally, Doxinate is not an antibiotic but a medicine to stop nausea and vomiting related to pregnancy. Your wife got well on her own, certainly not because of Doxinate.

122. What are the side-effects of levonorgestrel?

Q. What are the effects of levonorgestrel 1.5 mg on the normal menstrual cycle? I took the drug 40 hours after coitus and on the 5th day, bleeding occurred. Is there any chance of pregnancy after bleeding? Can it disturb the normal menstrual cycle?

A. There are no permanent side-effects. Sometimes there is a delay in resumption of menstruation (by more than 7 days) and/or spotting but it does not last very long. There is no effect on future fertility.

123. Will taking Zocon kit have a harmful effect on the fetus?

Q. I am 7 months pregnant and suffering from vaginal infection. My gynaecologist suggested that I take Zocon kit. Instead of taking 1 tablet at a time, I consumed the whole kit (consisting of 4 tablets) twice. After having the medicine I had severe nausea and felt very sleepy. My gynaecologist said that I took an extra dose and therefore I should take rest. Will this cause any harm to my fetus? What are the side-effects?

A. Zocon kit is the brand name: it contains three medicines: azithromycin, fluconazole and two tablets of secnidazole.

You can consume all the medicines of one kit at a time (except fluconazole since you are expecting). There will not be much problem even if you have taken double the dose except fluconazole tablets, which are not supposed to be prescribed to women during pregnancy at all.

Fluconazole in high doses is contraindicated in the first trimester of pregnancy, as it is a category C drug. Animal studies have shown it is fatal to the fetus. There are a few case reports of high-dose fluconazole taken in the first trimester for treatment of fungal infection in the mother, and infants born with congenital anomalies. Studies of its use at low doses and for short durations for the treatment of vaginal candidiasis indicate that such use is not associated with an increased incidence of congenital malformations, abortions or other adverse effects, and is therefore not necessarily an indication for termination of pregnancy. At 7 months, it can be given provided the benefit of using it outweigh the small risk at this time.

It is best to use miconazole or clotrimazole ointment or cream for *Candida* vaginitis during pregnancy. Miconazole should not be used vaginally if the membranes are ruptured (leakage of water). Untoward side-effects of miconazole cream are rare and include vaginal itching, burning and cramps.

Metronidazole is best avoided in the first trimester of pregnancy and also at other times. It is a category B drug. For treatment of *Trichomonas* infections, one can use clotrimazole vaginal tablets instead of metronidazole. As metronidazole is excreted in breast milk, it should not be taken by nursing mothers. Alternatively, one can take a single dose of 2 g for 1 day (for the treatment of *Trichomonas* vaginitis) and defer breastfeeding by 48 hours. At the same time, there are several reports of metronidazole use in all stages of pregnancy without adverse effects on the fetus. Accidental use in the first trimester is not an indication for termination of pregnancy. However, as it is fatal to the fetus in rodents, and reports in humans are insufficient, it is best avoided.

124. Will Duoluton-L have any adverse effects on pregnancy?

Q. I had my last period 2 months ago and the bleeding ended normally in 5 days. I was scheduled to have my period again last month, but it did not happen. I think I got pregnant, but I did not confirm it. Since I did not have periods that month, I began taking Duoluton-L. I have completed the course of 21 tablets today. Now I am worried whether I was pregnant and have lost the baby due to the medication. If I am pregnant, will the medicine prove risky for the pregnancy?

A. Duoluton-L is not allowed to be taken by women who are either pregnant or suspected to be pregnant. Due to ethical reasons, it is not possible to conduct clinical trials to determine the effect of the medicine in pregnant women. However, inadvertent intake of oral contraceptives (OCs) such as Duoluton-L in early pregnancy has neither affected the fetus nor caused any birth defects. You should be examined by a doctor to rule out any contraindications for the pills.

One point to remember is not to start a second packet unless you have your menses.

I assume that the pills have been taken regularly; therefore the chances of pregnancy are remote. However, I recommend that the fresh pack of pills should not be taken if your period does not start till 7 days after the last pill or if you have a bleed which is less than half of your usual amount. In such an event, you should be examined to rule out a pregnancy or an adverse effect of the OC.

Studies have not found any association between exposure in early pregnancy to OCs and congenital malformations – general, cardiac, limb or genital. However, the duration of exposure is neither mentioned nor consistent. Most of the contraceptive pills (including Duoluton-L) contain 19-nortestosterone derivatives as progestins. These progestins have been associated with masculinization of the exposed female fetus in women who took these drugs at higher doses, for reasons other than contraception.

In light of these facts, it is better that you have the pregnancy terminated (if confirmed), rather than live for 9 months with the anxiety. You must remember that even a 3-D ultrasound does not pick up all the abnormalities. Additionally, should the baby be born with a malformation (not related to the OC), you will always feel guilty.

125. Is taking ofloxacin harmful during pregnancy?

Q. I cut my toe with glass and was given Taracid (ofloxacin) 200 mg. At that time I didn't know that I was pregnant, which is about 7 weeks now. The conception might have happened while I was taking the antibiotic. My foot was swollen for a month and I was given antibiotics. I went for an ultrasound and the heartbeat of the fetus is all right. Will the antibiotic be harmful for my baby?

A. Good clinical practice demands that no drug (that is not permitted for use during pregnancy) should ever be prescribed to women of the reproductive age group, who or their sexual partners are not using contraception/condoms. If it becomes imperative to prescribe such a drug then a test should be done to exclude pregnancy.

Because of obvious ethical reasons, it is never possible to conduct clinical trials in humans to see if a drug would or would not cause fetal toxicity. However, reports on the inadvertent use of ofloxacin during pregnancy have not shown any adverse effects.

Besides, you would have consumed no more than 400 mg a day of ofloxacin, which comes to 8 mg per kg of your body weight. Animal studies have shown that such a dose does not have any adverse effect on late fetal development.

Since the ultrasound is normal, there is apparently no problem. As an abundant precaution, one should undergo ultrasonography at regular intervals.

Ofloxacin is a category C drug. The dose, duration, and time (week of pregnancy) of exposure of the drug should all be taken into account while calculating the risk of a drug. If a woman is not using contraceptives and is likely to become pregnant in the cycle when she requires antibiotic therapy (e.g. cuts, urinary infection, diarrhoea, etc.), a doctor should prescribe those that are proven to be safe during early pregnancy. This practice will save a lot of complications and anxieties for the pregnant woman, her family, as well as the prescribing doctor, should the woman later test positive for a pregnancy.

126. Is it safe to conceive if one is on aminosalicylic acid?

Q. I have been married for more than 2 years. I have been suffering from ulcerative colitis for the past 6 months and have had a relapse as well. Currently I am on medication, both allopathic and homeopathic. I have taken a total of three courses of steroids for one month each. I am in the last week of the last course of steroids. Apart from this I am also taking 5-aminosalicylic acid tablets 400 mg thrice a day as long-term treatment (from 6 months to 1 year). I want to conceive now, but I am not sure whether I'll have a safe pregnancy because of the long-term medication. My diet is without milk, fibre, fruits and vegetables. Please advise.

A. Generally, the use of 5-aminosalicylic acid (more commonly called mesalazine) for eight weeks results in remission of ulcerative colitis; hence I do not know why you are using it for 6 months or a year.

Mesalazine is a salicylate (just like aspirin). Even though data in humans on its use during pregnancy and breastfeeding are not available, it is not permitted to be used during the last weeks of pregnancy.

There is a small theoretical risk that mesalazine may produce premature closure of a vital passage in the heart (called the ductus arteriosus), may cause impairment of the renal (kidney) system in the fetus and may prolong labour and delay birth.

It is recommended that breastfeeding be discontinued during the use of mesalazine by the mother since the drug is excreted in the mother's milk.

A good nutritious diet, adequate in vitamins and minerals, is recommended so that the baby is not deprived of the same. However, this can be taken care of by taking supplements.

Ulcerative colitis that is quiescent at conception can relapse during pregnancy in about 30% of women. Half of the women with active disease at conception worsen during pregnancy. Therapy is the same as in the non-pregnant state. Maintenance with 5-aminosalicylic acid is continued and relapses require corticosteroids.

The outcome of pregnancy in women with ulcerative colitis seems to be controversial. In a review of 2398 pregnancy outcomes published since 1965, Modigliani (2000) concluded that there are no adverse pregnancy outcomes as compared to the general population. However, the report of Kornfeld and colleagues (1997) was contrary to this and showed an increased incidence of abortion, preterm labour and stillbirth. When colitis worsens during pregnancy, the cause may be psychogenic; hence reassurance and counselling are an important part of the management. Anaemia and nutritional deficiencies need to be corrected aggressively. You need to be under the care of an experienced gastroenterologist and obstetrician and should be registered for delivery in a tertiary centre.

127. Can Meprate lead to complications if taken during pregnancy?

Q. My wife happened to consume Meprate 10 mg tablets (twice a day for 5 days) in the 3rd and 4th weeks of pregnancy. The doctor prescribed it for getting normal periods, since the pregnancy test proved negative at that time. But later it was discovered that she was already pregnant. Now the fetus is 7 weeks old. I found that these tablets are not safe during pregnancy

and can harm the fetus by causing abnormality of the genitals. What are the risks involved and what should be done to minimize this risk? Is it safe to have the baby?

A. Meprate is the brand name of a medicine called medroxyprogesterone. It is used for

- Endometriosis
- Contraception
- Dysfunctional uterine bleeding
- Certain type of cancer

Hence I do not know why it was used for an unapproved indication. Good clinical practice demands that Meprate be given only in the first five days of menstruation (whether regular or irregular).

Pregnancy tests may be wrong. False-negative results do occur with urine tests, especially if it is not an early morning first sample and if it is an early pregnancy, and if the pregnancy test kit is not stored at the recommended temperature. A blood test for hCG is more sensitive for diagnosing early pregnancy, but it is 10 times more expensive than the urine test.

My choice in similar instances is Duphaston (dydrogesterone) which does not have any deleterious effect on the baby, if the woman later tests positive for pregnancy. Duphaston is again costlier than Meprate.

Meprate can cause toxicity to the fetus and malformation of organs, particularly genital abnormalities. It can also lead to virilization of a female baby (unwanted hair, etc.).

It is very difficult to quantify the possibility of malformation. According to one study the possibility of genital abnormality in a male fetus can be 10–16 per 1000 male births.

Since the risk is not unacceptably high, your wife can, if you both decide, continue with the pregnancy but do periodic, frequent ultrasound scans and other tests to make sure that everything is all right. On the other hand, any risk for congenital malformations, however small, is sufficient indication for a termination of pregnancy.

128. Can Buta-Proxyvon be safely consumed in pregnancy?

Q. My wife is undergoing hormone treatment for pregnancy. As the follicles are developed, we were asked to be in touch for four days. After two days,

she had headache and she took a pain killer by the name of Buta-Proxyvon. Will this have any adverse affect on the pregnancy?

A. Buta-Proxyvon is a combination product not meant for headache. Moreover, it is a 'prescription-only' medicine indicated for rheumatic disorders and should neither be bought nor used without a doctor's prescription. Your wife could have taken a simple analgesic such as Crocin (paracetamol) for headache.

Of the three ingredients in Buta-Proxyvon, diclofenac and dextropropoxyphene are not allowed during pregnancy. In case your wife does become pregnant, you should do frequent tests even though the chances of a congenital defect are quite small.

129. Can hydroxyurea lead to complications if taken during pregnancy?

Q. I am 22 years old and suffering from sickle ß-thalassaemia. I have been on treatment with hydroxyurea for nearly 2 years. I read an article on hydroxyurea for patients with sickle cell anaemia. I understand that there is huge risk for an unborn child. I missed my cycle last month and on testing found the serum beta hCG to be positive today. I am scared that the conception occurred during treatment. I had stopped taking the medicine from the day I missed my period. What is the effect of this treatment during pregnancy? What are the chances of my delivering a normal baby? What should I look for while taking a blood test?

A. Hydroxyurea has been found to be toxic to the fetus in animals. Data on use during human pregnancy is limited. However, clinical reports in humans show that the potential of fetal adverse effects is not very high, especially in first-trimester exposures, and no major malformation is described. There are reports of increased risk of intrauterine growth retardation and premature infants mainly in second-trimester use. (Majority of reported patients were on hydroxyurea due to myeloproliferative disorders, hence these complications can be due to the mother's primary condition rather than due to use of hydroxyurea.) My opinion is that such accidental first-trimester exposure should not be an indication for termination of pregnancy.

130. Are hMG and hCG safe during pregnancy?

Q. My wife has taken an hMG injection to get pregnant. Now, she is pregnant and in the 2nd month. She had some bleeding for which the doctor advised her to take Profasi 5000 IU injections once a week for 12 weeks of her pregnancy and Duphaston 10 mg twice a day for 12 weeks. I want to know the side-effects due to these hormones. Now, she is 11 weeks pregnant with no complaints of spotting or pain. The ultrasound too is normal. Please answer in detail about the possible side-effects on the baby and the mother. Also, she has dry cough. Can she take any allergy medicine or cough syrup?

A. Human menopausal gonadotrophin (hMG) is not indicated in pregnancy; human chorionic gonadotrophin (hCG) can be given in pregnancy – it is safe and is advisable in cases of proven progesterone deficiency. Instead of this, better option is to use micronized progesterone (Microgest) and Duphaston.

There are several cough medications that are safe in pregnancy. These would best be prescribed after thoroughly examining the patient's chest and paranasal sinuses. For this, please consult a family physician and inform him/her about the duration of the pregnancy.

131. Which antibiotics are safe during pregnancy?

Q. I am 12 weeks pregnant and my gynaecologist recently did a urine culture. The results showed that I have a bladder infection, for which she prescribed Augmentin (twice a day for 2 weeks). She said that the drug was safe, but I am not completely satisfied. Is this drug really safe? Will it do any harm to my baby? Is it true that baby girls tend to kick more or earlier than boys?

A. Women in the childbearing years are commonly treated with antibiotics and other antimicrobial medications. In pregnancy, the issue of which medication to use comes up frequently, whether for a bladder infection or other conditions. In general, every medication is assigned to a category (A, B, C, D, or X) based on how safe or risky it is to use during pregnancy. Only a few medications fall into category A, which means that human studies have shown no evidence of fetal harm in the first trimester or later in pregnancy. Most antibiotics are in category B, which means that there is no known association with birth defects or other pregnancy-related complication and the drug is probably safe. These include amoxicillin, ampicillin, augmentin (amoxicillin clavulanate), nitrofurantoin and cephalosporins. Others are in category C, meaning that either there is not enough information or there are some concerns arising from animal studies, but no confirmation of problems such as birth defects in humans. These include co-trimoxazole and trimethoprim, ciprofloxacin. Category D drugs are not safe and include tetracycline, doxycycline and sulpha drugs.

Tests and safety

132. Can I conceive the same month I underwent an X-ray?

Q. We have been trying to conceive for the past 12 months. The doctor suggested an X-ray to check if there was any problem in the uterus or the tubes. Everything was found to be all right. We did an X-ray on the 6th day after my periods. Is it all right to try for the baby in this month? In case I conceive this month, will there be any problem to the baby due to the X-ray?

A. It is completely safe to have a hysterosalpingogram or HSG (X-ray of the uterus and tubes using a contrast dye) in the first ten days of the menstrual cycle. The day the period starts is counted as the first day of the cycle. It is, therefore, completely safe for the baby to be conceived this month. Since the tubes get washed out during the X-ray procedure, there is a better chance of conceiving this month.

However, I would advise abstinence for at least 10 days after the HSG, as the woman is more likely to contract a pelvic infection due to vaginal intercourse immediately following a procedure. If the tubes have been opened due to the washing effect, they will remain open.

133. Why was my sac empty on ultrasound?

Q. 2 months ago, I had my periods for almost two weeks, which then stopped, but the severe abdominal cramps continued. My periods remained normal after that. I had a pregnancy test, which was negative. My doctor scheduled me for an ultrasound 4 weeks later, which showed an empty sac. I am rescheduled for another to see if anything appears, as they say it may be

too early to tell if a fetus is present. I am looking for a second opinion as to why the pregnancy test was negative. What does an empty sac mean? Should I be concerned? If there is no fetus present, what happens to this sac? Do I need medication to abort if there is no fetus present? Please advise.

A. An empty sac could be a very early pregnancy or a kind of abortion where the fetus does not develop. If this is confirmed, then you need to undergo abortion (cleaning of the uterus) which can be done with medicine or by surgery or by a combination of the two methods. The choice depends upon various factors including how big your uterus is, whether or not you have medical problems, allergy to certain drugs, etc.

The pregnancy test (if done on the urine) can be false negative if the sensitivity of the kit is not high, or the kit has not been stored at the recommended temperature. It can also be negative if you had an ectopic pregnancy (pregnancy outside the uterus), which has been disturbed. In your case, according to the ultrasound report, this is not so.

It is best to correlate the ultrasound findings with the clinical findings and the blood beta-hCG test. Your obstetrician will be the best person to guide you. Too many opinions (without examination) can, at times, do more harm than good.

134. Is a chest X-ray safe during pregnancy?

Q. I need to have a chest X-ray for Australian immigration but I am 23 weeks pregnant. So far, by the grace of God, everything is going smoothly. This is my first pregnancy. Is it safe to have a chest X-ray at this stage? My doctors, sonologist and radiologist have given me mixed answers, which has confused me. My immigration has already been delayed and it is like the last step for the case to be finalized. Please let me know if I can go through an X-ray to rule out TB.

A. It is best to inform the immigration authorities regarding the pregnancy. If their doctor still insists on getting the chest X-ray done, it can be done with an appropriate lead shield for the abdomen. These are routinely available in most X-ray clinics.

135. Is it safe to pass through metal detectors during pregnancy?

Q. I am 27 weeks pregnant. I will be travelling to India for my delivery. Is it safe to pass through metal detectors at the airport?

A. I would recommend you inform the staff at the check-in counters regarding your pregnant state and/or doubly check with the staff at the security check points regarding the safety of your being exposed to these machines. In case of doubt regarding the type of machines installed, the authorities usually limit the security check of a pregnant woman to only a manual 'hand check', without using any machines or gadgets.

136. Is exposure to microwave harmful during pregnancy?

Q. Is it safe to be exposed to the kitchen microwave during pregnancy?

A. Heavy exposure to electromagnetic waves or microwave emissions has been linked to reduced fertility in men.

Although it is impossible to prove that there is no risk for a developing fetus, research is very reassuring about ordinary exposure to low-level emissions, such as those produced by small appliances, e.g. a kitchen microwave.

137. Is the use of a cell phone harmful during pregnancy?

Q. I am a 34-year-old woman. I suffered from hyperprolactinaemia and was treated with bromocriptine tablets for a couple of years. Last year I got married and stopped taking the medicine but could not conceive. I consulted an obstetrician and he advised me to take bromocriptine for 3 months. While taking the medicine I got pregnant. It is now 2 months since I became pregnant. I plan to keep a cell phone but am afraid to use it as I have heard that hyperprolactinaemia is due to adenomas in the pituitary gland. Please advise – is it safe to use a mobile phone with hyperprolactinaemia?

A. Unless you have an existing tumour, which was causing the hyperprolactinaemia, you do not need to worry about the pregnancy or the cell phone making it worse. The cell phone will definitely not give rise to a brain tumour, as this seems to be the fear apparent from your query. There are many warning studies on the use of a cell phone but no adverse effects have been proved. As of today, a cell phone is considered safe in pregnancy. If you need to use it for work or normal communication you can and should use the cell phone. However, it is best to limit the usage of cell phones, as the distraction caused by talking while driving or working at home can lead to avoidable accidents.

I would like to know what the level of prolactin was in your blood when you started treatment and whether you are continuing bromocriptine after you became pregnant, also, whether the reason for the raised prolactin level was ever diagnosed before you became pregnant.

138. Is it safe to be near an MRI scanner during pregnancy?

Q. I am 10 weeks pregnant. I work in a firm which manufactures MRI scanners. I don't have to go near the scanner but I sit close to the room where the lab is. Is my baby safe and will this have any adverse effect on my baby?

A. It has been tested, tried and found to be safe if you are adjacent to an MRI magnet, even in pregnancy. In your case, you are outside the MRI room, which is completely sealed off. So you are definitely not affected by the MRI machine. However, in any case, you should inform the centre in-charge about your pregnancy.

Insurance

139. What is the 9-month waiting clause for maternity cover?

Q. My wife and I are covered under a group mediclaim policy bought by my employer. There is a clause of a 9-month waiting period for a maternity claim. I was explained that I cannot claim for maternity hospitalization until I have completed 9 months with the employer. I had completed 7 months and 3 weeks at the time of her hospitalization. My wife had an elective caesarean section because of breech presentation of the fetus. Can I at least claim the part of the expenses incurred for surgery only, since it was not a normal delivery? What could be the way to claim at least some part? Please advise.

A. The reason for the 9-month waiting clause is as follows: Insurance is taken/given for an unforeseen/unpredictable event that may happen in future. In case a woman is already pregnant when the maternity cover is granted then the logic of unforeseen/unpredictable does not hold good. Hence a claim is not accepted.

The method used in such cases is to check the date of the last menstrual period (LMP). In case the LMP was before the date the cover was taken then the claim is denied, but in case the LMP was after the cover was incepted, the claim thus arising is payable under the terms of the policy.

Therefore, you need to check two things: (a) The cover inception date for your family, which your office will be able to give you, and (b) check with your wife's doctor on the LMP date. If the date of cover inception is before the LMP then your claim is payable in full amount.

Health insurance rules should be checked with the respective insurance company. It is always better to directly discuss problems regarding claims with the insurance company.

140. Is there any health insurance policy which covers pregnancy?

Q. I would like to know whether any health insurance companies exist in India, which cover pregnant women, including charges of hospitalization in case of a caesarean delivery.

A. Individual medical insurance policies do not provide for maternity benefits (normal or caesarean) under the policy terms. But in case a group policy is issued, maternity benefits can be provided on payment of extra premium. A group policy is issued when there is a pre-defined group, viz. employees in an organization, credit card customers/account holders of a particular bank, etc. You may find out in case such a policy is available for your organization.

141. Why does insurance for pregnancy exist only under group policy?

Q. I am interested in taking a pregnancy Mediclaim policy. I have gone through the internet and the only information I have gathered is that insurance for pregnancy is not available for individuals. It only exists under group insurance. What do I do?

A. The reason why you want to take a medical insurance cover for pregnancy is obvious. You are planning to have your expenses covered for a planned delivery in the near future. Incidentally, insurance companies have the same fear as well, i.e. individuals who expect to claim are more keen on taking a policy than others, technically sometimes also referred to as adverse selection. Thus, no insurance company would like to provide a maternity cover. In a group policy, since the number of people covered is large, the risk is spread more evenly and widely, therefore, the probability of a claim is also reduced. I would recommend that you look for a group which offers a maternity cover and try to become a part of it, though finding such a group would undoubtedly be difficult since such groups are rarely open to individuals. Generally, a group would include an employer–employee group, credit card holders, bank customers, etc.

Abnormal pregnancy

- Abortion
- Miscarriage
- Complications during pregnancy
- Ectopic pregnancy
- Multiple pregnancy
- Pre-eclampsia and eclampsia
- Stillbirth

- Abortion and miscarriage
- High-risk pregnancy
- Problems of the fetus
- Placental abnormalities

Abortion

Abortion is the termination of pregnancy by any method (spontaneous or induced) before the fetus is viable (less than 20 weeks of pregnancy) and capable of surviving independently.

Induced abortion

Out of almost 35 million abortions which take place annually in the world, more than half of them are illegal and are performed by untrained, unskilled personnel under highly unhygienic conditions.

Abortion in the first trimester of pregnancy (up to 12 weeks)

Surgical methods

This is done by cervical dilatation, followed by evacuation of uterus or by using menstrual aspiration (MR).

Medical methods

Prostaglandins are the main group of drugs used nowadays. These can be taken orally or through injection intramuscularly/intravenously, or vaginally. These drugs are used either alone or in combination with other drugs.

- *Methotrexate–misoprostol method:* A woman receives an injection of methotrexate. She returns after 5–7 days for insertion of suppositories of misoprostol into her vagina.
- *Mifepristone–misoprostol method:* Mifepristone, also known as RU-486, is an antiprogesterone. A woman takes a dose of mifepristone and returns after 5–7 days for insertion of suppositories of misoprostol into her vagina.

Risks

- Mifepristone, methotrexate and misoprostol cause nausea and diarrhoea.
- Incomplete abortion may require surgical evacuation.
- Heavy bleeding may continue up to 7 days.

Abortion in the second trimester of pregnancy

In the second trimester of pregnancy, medical methods are preferred for abortion rather than surgical methods because of the risks involved. An early diagnosis of pregnancy with early termination is safer in the second trimester.

Methods of second trimester abortion (13–20 weeks) are explained below.

Medical methods

- *Ethacradine lactate:* This drug is introduced using a sterile catheter through the vagina into the uterine cavity and placed behind the pregnancy sac. This procedure is not painful. A maximum of 150 ml is instilled in the uterine cavity. It takes 48–72 hours to abort. The procedure is safe, cheap and easily available. To hasten the abortion, ethacridine can be used along with prostaglandin or oxytocin (a naturally available drug to increase uterine contractions).
- *Prostaglandin:* PG-E2, a gel of prostaglandin, is inserted into the cervix at the clinic and the patient is asked to lie down for about half an hour and then allowed to go home. The following morning, the pregnant woman is put on a drip of oxytocin intravenously, in the hospital. Complete abortion is usually achieved within 24 hours.
- *Misoprostol:* It can be given orally or inserted vaginally. About 24 hours later two tablets of mifepristone are given. The uterus contracts causing cramps followed by expulsion of the fetus. The cramps and the bleeding stop after the products have been expelled.
- *Others:* Drugs, such as urea, hypertonic saline, glucose, which are introduced into the pregnant sac, have all been discarded in favour of the above-mentioned methods.

The above medical methods require hospitalization for up to 3 days.

Risks

- Infection
- Increased bleeding
- Retained products may need surgical evacuation.

Surgical methods

Anaesthesia

General anaesthesia can be given depending on the pain threshold/ apprehension of the patient.

Procedure

Aspirotomy: This procedure is similar to the one done for first trimester abortion. This method can be employed when the woman is 13–20 weeks pregnant. Prostaglandins might be used to help in dilatation of the cervix.

Hysterotomy: It is a major surgery, similar to a caesarean section, where the abdomen is opened. In hysterotomy, the uterus is opened and the contents of the uterus are removed directly under vision. At times hysterotomy may be necessary because of failure of medical induction during the second trimester.

Hysterectomy: In this method, the uterus along with the pregnancy is removed *in toto*.

What is the Indian Medical Termination of Pregnancy (MTP) Act?

To avoid the misuse of induced abortions, laws have been enacted all over the world so that only qualified gynaecologists/obstetricians can perform MTPs for definite indications at approved clinics or hospitals. The Medical Termination of Pregnancy Act, 1971 was revised in 1975.

It lays down the conditions under which a pregnancy can be terminated and the people and places authorized to do so.

Indications for abortions under the MTP Act are:

1. When a pregnant woman has a serious disease and continuation of the pregnancy could endanger her life. Diseases include:
   - Heart disease
   - Severe hypertension
   - Uncontrolled vomiting during pregnancy
   - Cancer of the cervix or breast
   - Diabetes mellitus with eye complications (retinopathy)
   - Epilepsy
   - Psychiatric disorder.

2. Where the continuation of pregnancy could lead to substantial risk to the newborn causing serious physical or mental problems such as:
   - Chromosomal abnormalities
   - Rubella (German measles) infection in the mother during the first trimester
   - Congenital abnormalities in earlier births
   - Rh iso-immunization
   - Exposure of the fetus to irradiation
   - Pregnancy resulting from rape
   - Conditions where the socioeconomic status of the mother (family) hampers the progress of a healthy pregnancy and the birth of a healthy child
   - Failure of contraception, irrespective of the method used (natural, barrier or hormonal).

Consent

Married: The woman's written consent is required; husband's consent not necessary

Unmarried and over 18 years: Her own written consent

Below 18 years or mentally unstable: Written consent of guardian

Consent assures the clinician performing the procedure that the woman:

- has chosen abortion of her own free will.
- has been informed about all her options.
- has been counselled regarding the procedure (risks involved and care to be taken following it).

Who are the person(s) qualified to do MTP?

- A qualified registered medical practitioner who has assisted in at least 25 MTPs.
- A house surgeon who has completed 6 months' posting in Obstetrics and Gynaecology.
- A person who has a diploma/degree in Obstetrics and Gynaecology.
- A doctor with a minimum of 3 years of practice in Obstetrics and Gynaecology if registered before the enactment of the MTP Act, 1971.
- A doctor with a minimum of one year of practice in Obstetrics and Gynaecology if registered on or after the date of commencement of the Act.

Note: Whenever the pregnancy exceeds 12 weeks but is less than 20 weeks, the opinion of two registered medical practitioners (obstetricians) is mandatory before deciding on an MTP.

What are the approved places where MTP can be performed?

Any institution licensed by the Government to perform MTP is an approved MTP centre. The certificate issued by the Government has to be prominently displayed at a site readily visible to persons visiting the place.

Why is there a need for counselling?

Counselling is normally done by the attending doctor with the aim of helping the pregnant woman reach a decision as to the need for continuation or termination of the pregnancy and to resolve it in the direction that she chooses.

The purpose of counselling is to:

- Relieve the anxiety of the patient who intends to undergo the abortion.
- Provide information about the methods, safety and risks.

- Screen for guilt, or any psychiatric ailment.
- Help the patient understand and cope with her feelings.
- Help her to prevent a future unplanned pregnancy.

Serious complications arising from abortions before 13 weeks are rare. About 89% of the women who have abortions are less than 13 weeks pregnant. Of these women, 97% report no complications; 2.5% have minor complications that can be handled in the OPD or abortion facility; and less than 0.5% require some additional surgical procedure and/or hospitalization. Complication rates are higher for abortions performed between 13 and 20 weeks. General anaesthesia, which is sometimes used in abortion, carries its own risks.

In addition to the duration of the pregnancy, important factors that affect the possibility of complications include:

- Technical expertise of the provider;
- Risks due to anaesthesia;
- General health of the woman; and
- Method employed.

What are the complications from a legal abortion?
Possible complications from a surgical abortion procedure include:

- Blood clots accumulating in the uterus, requiring another suctioning procedure – required in less than 1% of cases;
- Infections, most of which are easily identified and treated if the woman carefully observes instructions – occur in less than 3% of cases;
- A tear in the cervix, which can be repaired with stitches – occurs in less than 1% of cases;
- Perforation in the wall of the uterus and/or other organs, which might heal on its own or might require surgical repair or, rarely, hysterectomy – occurs in less than 0.5%–1% of cases;
- Missed abortion, which does not end the pregnancy and requires the abortion procedure to be repeated – occurs in less than 0.5%–1% of cases;
- Incomplete abortion, in which tissue from the pregnancy remains in the uterus, and requires the procedure to be repeated – occurs in less than 1% of cases;
- Excessive bleeding due to failure of the uterus to contract, which might require blood transfusion – occurs in less than 1% of cases.

What are the warning signs of a post-abortion complication?
If a woman has any of the following symptoms after an abortion, she

should contact the facility that performed the abortion immediately.

- Severe pain
- Chills or fever with a temperature of 100.4 °F or more
- Bleeding that is heavier than the heaviest day of her normal menstrual period or that soaks through more than one sanitary pad in an hour
- Foul-smelling discharge from the vagina
- Continuing symptoms of pregnancy.

How can complications be prevented?
The risk of complications can be reduced by not delaying the abortion procedure. Once the woman is 6 weeks past the LMP, the earlier the abortion, the safer it is.

It is important to ask questions. Just as with any medical procedure, the more relaxed a woman is and the more she understands what to expect, the better and safer her experience will be.

In addition, any woman choosing abortion should:

- Find a good clinic with a qualified, licensed practitioner.
- Inform the practitioner of any health problems, current medications or allergies to medications or anaesthetics.
- Follow postoperative instructions.
- Return for a follow-up examination.

Miscarriage

A miscarriage or spontaneous abortion usually occurs before the 20th week of pregnancy. It is a natural way for the body to expel a fetus that is not expected to successfully grow into a baby. Miscarriage is fairly common since almost 10%–20% of all pregnancies are miscarried by the 12th week.

Most miscarriages that occur in the first trimester are due to abnormalities in the fetus. Miscarriages that occur in the second trimester are more often due to trauma to the mother. Miscarriage is different from abortion in that the latter is often used to refer to a pregnancy that is ended intentionally.

What are the various types of miscarriages?

Miscarriages may be classified according to the stage at which they occur and the nature of the miscarriage.

- Missed miscarriage – when the miscarriage has occurred but there are no visible signs and the remains have not been expelled from the uterus.
- Incomplete miscarriage – when the contents of the uterus have not been expelled completely. A dilatation and curettage (D&C) may have to be done to clean the uterus.
- Complete miscarriage – when the remains have been expelled from the uterus completely.
- Inevitable miscarriage – when the fetus is malformed and unable to continue as a viable pregnancy.
- Threatened miscarriage – when the signs of miscarriage are observed early in the pregnancy.
- Septic miscarriage – when infection occurs in the fetus before, during or after miscarriage.

How is it caused?

Though a miscarriage occurs when a pregnancy is not viable for continuation, there are some risk factors that predispose to miscarriage.

- Maternal age: The risk of a miscarriage increases with age. A woman is 20 times more likely to have a miscarriage at the age of 40 years than at 20.
- There is an increased risk of miscarriage if the woman has miscarried before or has had a stillborn child earlier.
- Women who suffer from diabetes, hypothyroidism or any other endocrine disorder are at high risk.
- Diseases such as systemic lupus erythematosus, uterine fibroids or endometriosis increase the risk.
- Conditions such as polycystic ovarian syndrome (PCOS), post-traumatic

stress disorder (PTSD), rubella, herpes, sexually transmitted infections (STIs), etc. also increase the risk.

- An abrupt fall in the body hormones might lead to a miscarriage.
- Excessive consumption of alcohol, caffeine and cigarettes increases the risk.
- Abnormality in the shape of the uterus or weakness of the organ can lead to a miscarriage.
- The risk of a miscarriage increases due to exposure to chemicals and other toxins.
- In some cases physical trauma or injury, can be the cause of miscarriage.

What are the signs?

The signs of a miscarriage are usually fairly obvious and can be easily discerned. Some of the common signs are:

- Abrupt vaginal bleeding in early pregnancy
- Abdominal cramps alternating with continuous stomach ache
- Pain in the lower back
- Painless expulsion of semi-solid matter from the vagina.

How is it diagnosed?

A blood and urine test confirms a pregnancy. The presence of a hormone called human chorionic gonadotrophin (hCG) in the body confirms pregnancy and its rising levels indicate the growth of a healthy fetus. Tests that may be done to check for an imminent miscarriage are:

- Complete blood count (CBC)
- White blood cell count to identify an infection
- Ultrasound to check for fetal movement and heartbeat
- Pelvic examination to check for traces of fetal tissue in the cervix or vagina.

What is the treatment?

Except in the case of a threatened miscarriage, the contents of the uterus have to be medically removed. A dilatation and curettage (D&C) is usually done by a gynaecologist/obstetrician to clean the uterus. The patient may be given antibiotics to prevent infection. Medications are given to help the uterus contract so that bleeding is reduced. If the miscarriage is caused due to Rh incompatibility, Rh immunoglobulins are given to such women to reduce the risk of miscarriage in subsequent pregnancies.

There may be some side-effects of treatment such as an allergic reaction to the anaesthesia, upset stomach, rashes on the body, abdominal cramps and vaginal bleeding. Fever may also occur in some women. The patient is usually sent home after regaining consciousness, but is advised complete bed rest for about 2 days. Exercise and intercourse are prohibited for some time depending on her general health.

How can it be prevented?

Miscarriages cannot usually be prevented but precautionary steps can be taken. Some of the guidelines are:

- The diet should be rich in vitamin B.
- Avoid caffeine and alcohol.
- Stop smoking completely during pregnancy.
- Sexual promiscuity may lead to sexually transmitted infections (STIs) that increases the risk of a miscarriage.
- Special care should be taken if the pregnant woman is suffering from a disease.

Complications during pregnancy

Pregnancies in which there is a risk to the mother, fetus or the newborn baby, before, during or after delivery, are called high-risk pregnancies.

Common abnormalities that affect pregnancy

- Spontaneous abortion (miscarriage)
- Ectopic pregnancy
- Hyperemesis gravidarum
- Placenta praevia
- Abruptio placentae
- Rh incompatibility (erythroblastosis fetalis)
- Multiple pregnancies
- Pre-eclampsia and eclampsia

Spontaneous abortion (miscarriage)

Termination of pregnancy that occurs before the 28th week is called abortion. When abortion is natural and not induced, it is called spontaneous abortion or miscarriage. If the pregnancy ends between the 28th and 40th week, it is not called an abortion, but premature labour since the baby is considered to be viable in the third trimester. The incidence of abortion is generally believed to be as high as 30% of all pregnancies.

Causes of miscarriage include:

- Abnormalities in the fetus
- Intrauterine death due to infections contracted by the mother (e.g. malaria, typhoid, dysentery, etc.) and effects of X-rays or drugs
- Abnormalities of the placenta
- Abnormalities of the mother's genital system.

Ectopic pregnancy

Pregnancy that occurs when the fertilized egg implants itself outside the uterus is called an ectopic pregnancy. Two kinds of ectopic pregnancies are common – tubal pregnancy (when the egg gets implanted in the fallopian tubes) and ovarian pregnancy (when implantation takes place in the ovaries).

- Tubal pregnancies often end in spontaneous abortion since the fallopian tubes do not have enough space for a fetus to grow. In such cases, the uterus also becomes enlarged and may look like a normal pregnant uterus of about 2 months. Women who have a blockage in one of the tubes are more prone to ectopic pregnancy. Also, women who have had surgery for reversal of tubal sterilization are also at an increased risk for tubal pregnancy.

- Ovarian pregnancies, though rare, are more difficult to detect than tubal pregnancies. In this, the sperm penetrates the egg before the latter has had a chance to come out of the ovary. Implantation takes place in the walls of the ovary.

Hyperemesis gravidarum

It is a condition characterized by excessive nausea and vomiting during pregnancy, which leads to weight loss. The pregnant woman remains dehydrated most of the time and has to be on medication. The patient may need to be hospitalized till the situation is brought under control. She is given liquid nutrition intravenously followed by a very light fluid diet. The patient is under continuous medical supervision and, in rare cases, the doctor may have to terminate the pregnancy. Usually, the pregnant woman is able to regain the lost weight once the condition is successfully treated.

Placenta praevia

It is a complicated medical condition where the placenta covers the opening of the cervix into the vagina. In most cases, an early ultrasound may detect a low-lying placenta. The situation usually resolves by itself as the uterus grows larger.

The condition may be detected by sudden and heavy painless vaginal bleeding towards the end of the second trimester. There may be danger to the life of the mother and the baby if the bleeding does not stop. In most cases of incessant bleeding, the baby is delivered by caesarean section if the pregnancy is beyond the 30th week. If the pregnancy is not in the last stages, the patient is advised complete bed rest and any kind of sexual arousal is avoided.

Abruptio placentae

It is a condition in which the placenta begins to separate from the wall of the uterus before the end of the pregnancy. It is a relatively rare condition and women with heart problems, high blood pressure and those who smoke are more at risk for developing a detached placenta.

The main symptom of the condition is bleeding and cramps in the abdominal region, the severity of which depends on the extent of dislocation. In mild cases, the patient can resume her normal routine after some days of bed rest. Adequate rest is the most effective treatment for mild-to-moderate cases. In case the bleeding is very severe, immediate delivery is required to prevent any harm to the mother and the baby.

Rh incompatibility (Erythroblastosis fetalis)

This condition is caused due to incompatibility of certain blood components of the mother and the baby. Also known as Rh incompatibility, there is destruction of the fetal blood cells due to antibodies transmitted from the maternal blood. The first child is usually normal and healthy. The effects are seen in subsequent children, when anti-D antibodies (against Rh-positive blood) are already present in the mother's body. The condition occurs when a woman with an Rh-negative blood group is impregnated by a man with an Rh-positive blood group and the fetus happens to be Rh-positive. The fetal blood causes antibodies to be generated in the mother's body, which may be transferred to and affect subsequent babies.

Treatment is aimed at improving the immunity of the mother's body. In some cases, fetus may have to be transfused within the uterus. If the pregnancy proceeds without much of a problem, the baby will deliver normally and the attending doctor will be prepared to transfuse blood in the newborn, if necessary.

Multiple pregnancies

Though not a complicated pregnancy in the strictest sense, multiple fetuses require more attention. Apart from competition for nutrition and space, multiple babies may be placed abnormally inside the uterus. In some cases, one baby may be head down (normal), while the other may be bottom down (breech baby). Some babies may also be entwined laterally (like a T).

Ectopic pregnancy

A pregnancy that takes place outside the uterus is called an ectopic pregnancy. In a normal pregnancy, the fertilized egg implants itself in uterine wall and the fetus grows there. In an ectopic pregnancy, the implantation can take place anywhere outside the uterus, in the fallopian tubes (tubal pregnancy), ovaries (ovarian pregnancy) or in the abdominal cavity.

Ectopic pregnancy is a complication that has to be medically terminated. Of the ectopic pregnancies, more than 97% take place in the fallopian tubes.

What are the causes?

It is caused due to the inability of the fertilized egg to travel to the uterus for successful implantation. This may be because of an abnormality of the fallopian tubes, which prevents the egg from travelling downwards. Women who have undergone tubal sterilization or who have had successful reversal of the sterilization are more likely to contract infections and are more at risk for ectopic pregnancies.

Other risk factors that may increase the chances of an ectopic pregnancy are:

- Previous ectopic pregnancy
- Pelvic inflammatory disease
- Infertility
- Abdominal injury
- Hormonal imbalance leading to impaired fallopian tube contraction
- Smoking
- Placement of an intrauterine device (like Copper-T).

What are the symptoms?

Some of the symptoms of an ectopic pregnancy may be the same as those which occur during a normal pregnancy, and thus may not be immediately discernible. These may include abdominal pain, vaginal bleeding, weakness and dizziness. They may also be accompanied by tenderness in the breasts, nausea, low back pain and stomach cramps. Occasionally there is major bleeding into the abdomen and the patient may present in a state of shock with a rapid pulse and low blood pressure.

How is it diagnosed?

Ectopic pregnancies are often difficult to diagnose. The first indication may be irregular periods. A pregnancy test that measures the level of the hormone human chorionic gonadotrophin (hCG) is able to discern whether the pregnancy is normal, in which case the hormone levels double every day, or ectopic in which case the rise in hCG levels do not follow this pattern.

Some other tests that may be done to make the diagnosis are white blood cell count, ultrasound examination and laparoscopy.

What is the treatment?
Treatment may be chemical or surgical. Chemical treatment involves drug therapy with methotrexate. It is a non-urgent form of treatment in which the fetus is dissolved without harming the tubes and the surrounding organs. The drug brings down the hCG levels in the blood thus nullifying the pregnancy. The hCG levels are brought down to zero within 4 weeks.

Surgery involves laparotomy that results in the removal of the fetus and other products of conception. The ruptured surrounding organs are also cleaned and repaired. The procedure requires a 5 cm incision in the abdominal wall through which the fallopian tubes are accessed. The ectopic pregnancy is then removed and the wound is closed.

What are the chances for future pregnancies?
There is a chance that the next pregnancy may also be ectopic. If one of the fallopian tubes is removed during surgery (salpingectomy), the chances of conception may be reduced. However, under supervision, pregnancy can be attempted again. Physical healing depends on the patient's general health.

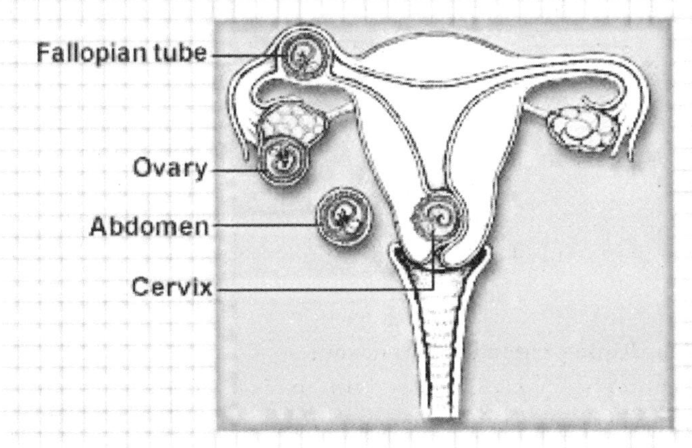

ECTOPIC PREGNANCY

Multiple pregnancy

A multiple pregnancy is one in which there is more than one fetus in the uterus. Multiple births are a relatively rare phenomena and only about 1 in 36 babies born is a pair of twins. Triplets or multiplets are even rarer. Multiple births have become more common since the availability of fertility treatments. This is because more than one fertilized egg is introduced into the uterus, leading to twin or triplet pregnancies.

Types of twins?

Fraternal twins: They are the most common type of twins. Fraternal twins are no more alike - genetically and in their looks - than any regular pair of siblings. Fraternal twins are formed when two separate eggs are fertilized by two different sperm. They share only the uterine space and the intrauterine environment. Fraternal twins may not be of the same sex and they may also not look alike. Fraternal twins are also called dizygotic.

Identical twins: Identical twins are born when the fertilized egg splits into two distinct entities in the early stages of cell division. The DNA and other genetic material is shared by the twins. They have the same genotype and phenotype, which means that they not only have a similar genetic make-up but also similar external characteristics. Identical twins share the same amniotic sac but have separate placentas. They are always of the same sex and are also called monozygotic.

Siamese or conjoined twins: A variation of identical twins, these twins are joined at one or the other body part. This is because of incomplete splitting of the fertilized egg during pregnancy leading to incompletely separated individuals. Siamese twins, like identical twins, look alike and are of the same sex. However, conjoined twins are joined at some point in their bodies and may also share some organs. Conjoined twins have been known to be joined from the head, chest, stomach and hips.

Mirror twins: They are a variation of identical twinning, these twins are mirror images of each other. They are extremely rare. Such twins have organs on the opposite sides, for example one twin will have the heart on the right side instead of the left and will be opposite handed to the other twin.

How is a multiple pregnancy diagnosed?

A multiple pregnancy is diagnosed with the help of a routine ultrasound. The doctor will check for the presence of two amniotic sacs and separate placentas in case of a multiple pregnancy. The mother's abdomen may also be larger than usual if she is carrying more than one baby.

Why do multiple pregnancies occur?

Multiple pregnancies usually occur by chance, but the probability may be more in women who have a family history of multiple pregnancies. They can also result from the fertility treatments that women undergo to increase their chances of pregnancy. Older mothers are more likely to have multiple births than younger ones. In some cases, certain medication cause the release of more than one egg which increases the chances of having a multiple pregnancy.

What are the complications?

There are some risks that multiple fetuses may be prone to:

- Preterm birth – multiple pregnancies usually do not reach full term and may need to be delivered by a caesarean section.
- Slow intrauterine growth of the babies due to sharing of all nutrients from the mother
- Birth defects
- Anaemia
- Complications of the amniotic sac, umbilical cord or the placenta
- Too much fluid in the amniotic sac
- Death of one or more fetuses.

What problems does the mother face?

The mother may also have to face certain problems in case of a multiple pregnancy. Some of these are:

- Excessive weight gain
- Conditions such as hyperemesis gravidarum
- Gestational diabetes
- Toxaemia of pregnancy (high blood pressure)
- Postpartum haemorrhage (excessive bleeding after delivery)

What are the precautions to be taken?

As soon as it is diagnosed that the woman is carrying multiple fetuses, she may be prescribed more rest than in a normal pregnancy. Extra care has to be taken during the pregnancy since the chances of a preterm birth are greatly increased. Also, the babies tend to be smaller than single babies. Frequent tests may be done to ensure the good health of the babies. Dietary modifications may be needed since the pregnant woman needs a larger amount of nutrition to meet her needs. It should be decided in advance whether the babies would be born vaginally or by a caesarean section. Any complication should be brought to the notice of the doctor.

Pre-eclampsia and eclampsia

Pre-eclampsia and eclampsia are conditions that occur during pregnancy and are associated with high blood pressure, loss of protein in the urine and swelling of the body. Pre-eclampsia is also called toxaemia of pregnancy, which may develop into eclampsia if it is complicated by fits. These conditions usually develop in the second half of pregnancy, though sometimes they develop shortly after delivery.

What are the causes?

The exact cause of this problem is not known. The disorder is triggered by one or more substances produced by the placenta (also known as the afterbirth), which induces a generalized reaction in the pregnant woman. One of the main features of this effect is a constriction of the small arteries of the body.

What are the symptoms?

- Rapid weight gain
- Swelling of the feet, ankles, hands and face
- Headache and dizziness
- Ringing in the ears
- Abdominal pain
- Decreased production of urine
- Nausea and vomiting
- A state of confusion

Who is at risk?

- Women who are pregnant for the first time
- Women who have a family history of such a problem
- Women who are 40 years old or more
- Women with pre-existing high blood pressure
- Obese women
- Women expecting twins or triplets

What are the complications associated with the problem?

- A very high blood pressure interferes with the placenta's ability to transfer oxygen and nutrients to the baby, resulting in a low birth weight baby with other developmental problems.
- Very high blood pressure can cause malfunctioning of the kidneys.
- There can be destruction of the red blood cells, disturbed liver function and a decrease in the number of platelets (blood cells that play a key role in the clotting process). A decreased platelet count can lead to uncontrollable bleeding during delivery.

- If the blood pressure is not kept under control it can lead to eclampsia wherein the woman develops fits leading to a decreased supply of oxygen to the baby. The placenta may also start to separate from the wall of the uterus.

How is it diagnosed?
A woman's blood pressure is always measured at every visit to the doctor and a record is maintained. If the diastolic (lower reading) blood pressure is found to be high (95 mmHg or more instead of the normal 80 mmHg) and/or the systolic (upper reading) is found to be 150–160 mmHg instead of the normal 120 mmHg or if there is protein in the urine as diagnosed by urine examination, the condition is called pre-eclampsia.

What is the treatment?
The treatment of pre-eclampsia is bed rest and as soon as the fetus has a good chance of survival outside the womb the doctor should decide on delivery. Careful monitoring of the blood pressure, weight and urine for protein is needed. Delivery can be induced in the following instances:

- The diastolic blood pressure increases from 80 mmHg (normal) to 100 or 110 mmHg and remains at that level consistently for a 24-hour period.
- Persistent or severe headache
- Pain in the abdomen
- Abnormal liver functions as diagnosed by tests
- Abnormal fetal heart rate.

How can it be prevented?
- There are no known preventive methods for this condition. An early diagnosis through regular visits to the doctor during pregnancy thus becomes important.
- Taking a calcium tablet daily during pregnancy may possibly decrease the risk of developing these disorders.

Stillbirth

Stillbirth is the death of the baby in the womb after 20 weeks of pregnancy. Stillbirth occurs in about 1 in 200 pregnancies. It is a tragic and heartbreaking experience, because it ends a pregnancy that was seemingly problem-free. In most of the cases, the loss is completely unexpected. About 14% of these deaths occur during labour and delivery, and the rest occur before labour begins.

What are the causes?

Stillbirths could be due to maternal, fetal, or uterine factors. Injuries, illnesses (such as toxaemia), infections, or catastrophic events (such as haemorrhage, or cardiac arrest) could affect both mother and child. Birth defects and growth abnormalities of the fetus can also occur. Uterine factors (such as placental detachment, placental obstruction, or restricted uterine growth) can prove dangerous to the fetus. Alcohol, drugs and tobacco use during pregnancy can cause stillbirth and infant death.

What are the signs?

The first sign of a problem that a pregnant woman notices, is that her baby has stopped moving and kicking. Stillbirth is usually diagnosed before birth by an ultrasound, and labour is generally induced. After delivery the baby and placenta are examined to help determine the cause of death. Even with exhaustive testing, in up to one-third of cases, the cause of stillbirth cannot be determined.

How is it diagnosed?

An ultrasound examination can confirm that the baby has died. The doctor then performs a few blood tests on the pregnant woman, which helps determine the cause of the death.

What is the treatment?

If there is no medical reason for immediate delivery, the couple can decide when they want to deliver the baby. In most cases, a woman undergoes labour within 2 weeks after the death. If a woman chooses to wait for labour to begin it poses little risk to her health. However, because of the emotional trauma of carrying a dead baby, most women choose to have induced labour. If the woman's cervix has not begun to dilate in preparation for labour, she is given vaginal suppositories to help prepare her cervix, followed by the hormone oxytocin (which is given through a vein), which stimulates uterine contractions. Generally, a caesarean is recommended only if a woman develops problems with labour and delivery. If labour does not begin within two weeks, doctors recommend inducing labour to avoid problems related to clotting of blood.

How is it prevented?

Stillbirths have declined significantly, over the past 20 years. This is mostly due to better treatment options available for certain conditions such as maternal high blood pressure and diabetes, which increases the risk of stillbirth. The incompatibility between the blood of the mother and the baby is an important cause of stillbirth. This can now be prevented by giving an Rh-negative woman an injection of immune globulin at 28 weeks of pregnancy, and again after the birth of an Rh-positive baby.

Women with high-risk pregnancies are carefully monitored during late pregnancy. Tests that monitor the fetal heart rate can often tell if the baby is in danger. Treatments are now available for this, which sometimes include early delivery that can be lifesaving. Today, women with well-controlled diabetes and high blood pressure face very little risk of stillbirth.

Doctors suggest that all pregnant women at high and low-risk should do a daily 'kick count' starting around 26 weeks of pregnancy. If a woman counts less than 10 kicks a day, or if she feels that the baby is moving less than usual, her doctor may recommend tests to determine fetal well-being (such as fetal heart rate monitoring and ultrasound). If the tests show that the baby could be in trouble, steps can be taken to prevent death.

Women should not smoke, drink alcohol or use drugs, as all these increase the risk of stillbirth and can create other complications. Women should report any vaginal bleeding to their consulting doctor immediately. Vaginal bleeding during the second half of pregnancy can be a sign of placental abruption. When the fetus is in trouble due to an abruption, a prompt caesarean delivery can be lifesaving.

A woman who has had a stillbirth in a previous pregnancy should be monitored carefully, so that all necessary steps can be taken to prevent another death.

What steps can one take?

One needs to consult a doctor immediately, if the baby's movements have decreased or stopped, or if there is bleeding from the vagina. High blood pressure or diabetes has to be monitored regularly and should be kept under control. One should follow doctor's advice and take any medication as directed. If one does have a stillbirth, one should allow oneself time to recover physically and emotionally from the pregnancy and delivery.

How to deal with the loss of a baby?

Most babies are born healthy. But, sometimes, something goes wrong and the baby dies. The death of an infant is, perhaps, the most difficult and wrenching tragedy any family can imagine. Besides the physical loss, there is an emotional loss and a loss of all that a new life promises. This is true whether the baby died as a newborn or before birth due to miscarriage, stillbirth or other reasons. Society has been slow to recognize that the impact on the parents can be the same regardless of when the loss occurred. Parents' grief over miscarriage is as valid and real as their grief over the loss of a full-term baby.

Parents never really 'get over' the loss of their baby. But they learn to live without his physical presence and, eventually, integrate the loss into their life's experience. It is important for parents who suffer the loss of a baby to realize that they can and will move through their grief. While grieving is a very individual experience, it also is a process that has a number of phases. Sometimes the phases overlap, some may be skipped, some repeated. Everybody deals with grief differently. There is no right or wrong way to grieve.

Abortion and miscarriage

142. How long does the body take to recover after a D&C?

Q. **I had a D&C done in my 3rd month of pregnancy as the growth of the child was not proper. How long does it take for recovery? What is the duration for taking rest? What foods should I avoid? I have slight bleeding only when I cough. Otherwise there is no continuous flow. How long will this bleeding continue?**

A. The body takes 6 weeks after a pregnancy or abortion to return to the normal pre-pregnancy state.

Usually, one week of rest is adequate. However, the period of rest advised depends upon any complication encountered during the dilatation and curettage (D&C) such as excessive bleeding, or any other pre-existing medical condition you may be suffering from.

You can take any food that constitutes a healthy diet, or whatever suits you. Avoid spicy and greasy foodstuffs – these aggravate the indigestion that usually occurs with antibiotic intake.

You can expect some bleeding for up to 1 week. Any bleeding which is more than two fully soaked sanitary towels per day is abnormal and you need to report it to your gynaecologist/obstetrician immediately. (*See also* page 136)

143. How does an incomplete abortion occur?

Q. **How does an incomplete abortion happen? What are its signs and symptoms? What follow up should be done?**

A. If a patient has spontaneous abortion, then a part of the fetus or products of conception may remain behind. It is then called an incomplete abortion.

Sypmtoms include excessive bleeding and pain in the abdomen. Routine blood tests are done as a follow up after an abortion. The patient will have to undergo D&C and is called for a check-up after 10 days. (*See also* page 136)

144. Why did I have an incomplete abortion?

Q. I had a myomectomy done 4 years ago and had an incomplete abortion last year after a course of Clomid. My report said that a single line enucleation was done of the fibroids in my womb. Do you think the embryo was unable to attach itself to the womb as a result of the residual mass? Can it attach itself to a surgery site on the residual mass? What is the best fertility treatment after myomectomy?

A. If you are unable to conceive (secondary infertility) after the last abortion, then you and your husband need to be investigated. As you have said that you conceived after treatment with Clomid, I suppose you have ovulatory dysfunction.

The cause of abortion depends upon the period of gestation at which it occurred. Sometimes, an abortion can occur if implantation of the fertilized egg occurs at a scarred site, due to ineffective placentation. However, there is no way of predicting where the implantation will occur, nor any method to diagnose whether or not it has implanted on the scarred site. (*See also* page 136)

145. Why did my baby die and when should we try for another baby?

Q. I am 31 years old and my wife is 28 years old. We got married last year and this month my wife delivered a stillborn baby. The doctors say that there was a blood clot, which is the reason for the death of the baby. My wife had high blood pressure on the day (160/90 mmHg) just before the delivery. What were the possible reasons for the death of the baby and when should we start our normal sexual life? When should we try for a pregnancy?

A. It is difficult to tell you the possible cause of death. Obviously, there was fetal anoxia (the fetus did not receive enough oxygen). I presume what the doctors meant was that there was antepartum haemorrhage (bleeding before the delivery of baby), and this was probably due to premature separation of the placenta. Your obstetrician is the best person to answer this question. I would be doing an injustice by trying to state the possible reasons; nor is it correct to do so without knowing the details of the sequence of events.

We do not advise sexual intercourse till at least 6 weeks after delivery. This interval may be prolonged depending upon the findings of examination at 6 weeks (postpartum check-up). One should also keep in mind the mental state of your wife, as the loss is hardest for the mother.

You should avoid a pregnancy for at least 6 months. Also, make sure her blood pressure is normal in the interval (non-pregnant) period, and ensure that all the possible tests have been done to ascertain the causes of the baby's death.

146. My wife had a miscarriage in her first pregnancy. What precautions should we follow in this one?

Q. My wife had a miscarriage last year in the 2nd month of pregnancy. She is pregnant once again. She should have frequent urination and a heavy feeling in her abdomen. She had these symptoms only for a few days but not now. We have not approached any doctor so far. Please tell me what care should we take and how to check that everything is normal.

A. Congratulations and very good wishes for a smooth pregnancy for your wife! Some women do have the problem of frequent urination in the early part of their pregnancy but this is not a hard and fast rule. What is highly recommended at this point is that you get a book titled *What to expect when you are expecting*. You can find the details of this in the medical publications section of www.doctorndtv.com. Meanwhile, here are a few important dos and don'ts: Your wife should start having folic acid tablets or capsules (Cobadex forte, Becosules, etc.) once a day, plenty of fruits and green vegetables, milk, egg, yoghurt, avoid carrying weights or doing any vigorous exercise for the time being, particularly in view of her earlier miscarriage. The first trimester is very important for the well-being of both the baby and mother. She requires regular check-ups by her obstetrician, so you should choose one now with whom you both are comfortable and who is attached to a good hospital where your wife's weight, blood tests, urine, blood pressure and fetal heart sounds can be periodically checked up and she can be given her anti-tetanus shots at the right time. (*See also* page 136)

147. Are 'over-the-counter' drugs safe for terminating a pregnancy?

Q. I have not yet consulted an obstetrician for my problem but a chemist gave

me two medicines for termination of pregnancy – norethindrone acetate and Beplex forte tablets manufactured by Sandoz. The chemist said that I will get my periods by the 4th day. I started taking these tablets since last night. I want to know if this method is safe. Will it help me in terminating my pregnancy? I didn't want to consult an obstetrician because nobody in my family and husband's family would agree to it. Please advise as soon as possible.

A. It is not only foolish but dangerous to consume 'prescription-only' medicines without a doctor's prescription. It is also illegal for chemists (most of whom are lay people owning a drug store without any professional qualification) to prescribe medicines. Norethindrone is not meant for termination of pregnancy. I suggest you immediately and urgently consult either a gynaecologist/obstetrician or an NGO like Marie Stopes Clinic or Family Planning Association of India, etc. to avoid getting into serious trouble.

It is important to note that you should fulfil the criteria specified by the Government of India (GOI) to undergo termination of pregnancy—be it medical or surgical. Majority of women seeking abortion are unaware of this. Every abortion has side-effects. It is the duty of the gynaecologist/obstetrician to ensure that the woman seeking abortion does indeed fulfil the conditions specified by the GOI. Otherwise, women would use abortion rather than contraceptives as a means of limiting family size. GOI has laid down this rule so that people do not misuse liberalization of abortion.

Medical abortion with tablets has to be done under the strict supervision of a qualified obstetrician. The guidelines drafted by the GOI and WHO have to be followed. Medical abortion with pills is recommended only for pregnancies up to 49 days from the last menstrual period. The success rate is approximately 97%. In case of failure, the pregnancy has to be terminated surgically. Therefore, medical abortion is not to be carried out in a woman who does not consent for surgical abortion in case of failure of the medical abortion. Also, intrauterine pregnancy should be confirmed before administering the pills, and the scan should be repeated after 14 days to confirm complete abortion. The woman should be willing to undergo emergency surgical abortion in case of incomplete abortion or heavy bleeding. (*See also* page 136)

148. Can I plan a pregnancy after miscarriage due to toxoplasmosis?

Q. Is it possible to have a safe pregnancy after a missed abortion due to a

positive test for *Toxoplasma gondii*? If one has completed a 3 months' course of spiramycin, are there any chances of abortion again or is it curable?

A. Yes, it is possible to have a safe pregnancy after previous miscarriage due to toxoplasmosis. The best thing is to periodically monitor *Toxoplasma* serology and monitor the fetus by ultrasound during the pregnancy. It is always better to be in touch with an experienced obstetrician to review the management and consider any intervention, if needed. The obstetrician can in turn liase with a local microbiologist or the lab which conducts these special serological tests and monitor the course of the pregnancy. A woman with chronic or latent infection prior to conception does not transmit the infection to the fetus. The extremely rare cases of congenital toxoplasmosis of babies born to women with chronic infection (less than 1% of all congenital toxoplasmosis cases), occur in women who are immunocompromised (e.g. those on heavy prolonged doses of steroids, chemotherapy for cancer and with HIV infection). (*See also* page 136)

149. What is the reason for continuous bleeding after an MTP?

Q. I underwent medical termination of pregnancy (MTP). The bleeding continued for 14 days and after an ultrasound examination, it was found that the termination had not been complete. The doctor gave me another pill to insert in the vagina and the bleeding lasted for 7 days. The next ultrasound showed that everything is okay and the bleeding stopped. However, it started again after 3 days. Is there something to worry about?

A. This is one problem with medical termination of pregnancy – bleeding is not predictable. I suppose you did have an ultrasound scan done before the MTP to ensure pregnancy was indeed within the uterus, and not outside (ectopic pregnancy). If repeat scan has shown complete abortion, then there is no worry. However, it is better to undergo an internal examination by your gynaecologist/obstetrician to make sure there is no evidence of infection (unlikely if you have not had sex in the intervening period). Also, sometimes it is better to get a serum beta hCG done and follow it up to ensure everything is all right. (*See also* page 136)

150. How can I prevent a miscarriage due to a positive ANA?

Q. My wife suffered a miscarriage; the cause of which the doctor said was the

presence of antinuclear antibodies (ANA) (we were planning an IVF). She weighted 75 kg and is 5.2 in height. We will make a second attempt soon but want to prevent a miscarriage. The doctor says my wife has to take steroids; could you please enlighten me on the process and side-effects of this?

A. ANA (antinuclear antibodies) is a test and not diagnosis of any disease. ANA is positive in a large number of disorders such as fibromyalgia, systemic sclerosis, systemic lupus erythematosus (SLE), iatrogenic (due to consumption of certain medicines), etc. If possible, it is always worthwhile to determine the cause of the presence of ANA. Steroids do kill antibodies and thus counter ANA. The details given by you are not sufficient for me to give you advice on their use in your wife's specific case. My concern is also the weight of the patient: at 72 kg and 5 feet 2 inches of height, she is already substantially overweight (in all probability due to hypothyroidism); steroids will increase the weight further. One has to see whether the side-effects are balanced by benefits.

151. Can I conceive if one fallopian tube has been removed?

Q. Six months ago, I was operated for an ectopic pregnancy in which my right fallopian tube was removed. I took AKT 4 tablets for 2 months. Now I am on Rifampin and Isoniazid capsules for uterine infection. I am 30 years old. When can I take a chance at pregnancy?

A. If the other tube is patent and free of adhesions, you have a fairly good chance of pregnancy through it. However, in case you fail to achieve a normal pregnancy in the required time-frame, *in vitro* fertilization (IVF) is always an option, though I would suggest adoption.

Tuberculosis was probably diagnosed at laparotomy and confirmed by pathological examination of the removed tube. The 'uterine infection' was probably diagnosed by pathological examination of the endometrial tissue. TB of the genital tract involves the fallopian tubes in nearly all cases. These tubes are usually functionally damaged despite full treatment. Intrauterine conception is rare in such cases, despite having one remaining tube. IVF is an option, provided the endometrium is functional, and there are not too many intrauterine adhesions (diagnosed by hysteroscopy). Antituberculous treatment (ATT) needs to be taken for a full 9 months. It is important to repeat the endometrial biopsy after 8–10 weeks of treatment to ensure that you are responding to the ATT.

High-risk pregnancy

152. Why did I have premature rupture of membranes?

Q. I lost a baby after a preterm delivery due to leakage of amniotic fluid at the end of the 28th week. The baby died after 42 days in the neonatal intensive care unit (NICU) due to sudden development of sepsis on the 35th day, which was not responsive to medicines. What could be the reason for the breach of membrane? I had a normal pregnancy except a slightly higher BP during the first trimester, which was controlled with alphadopa. I also had Profasi shots twice weekly, during the initial stages of pregnancy. Only two days before the breach occurred, I had an ultrasonography (USG) done, which showed no abnormalities. Now I am trying to conceive again. What precautions should we take this time? I have read about stitches during the 14th week to counter possible cervical incompetence. How is this done? Does it require surgery? I have also read that the growing bag is not big enough to hold the baby till the 9th month.

A. There are numerous reasons for premature rupture of membranes. The most important one is infection. There may not be any symptoms in the pregnant lady before the leakage. It may be difficult for a preterm baby born at 28 weeks to survive, and if he does, he can have delayed milestones, etc. Perhaps God has spared you and the baby of problems that would have occurred later.

An incompetent cervix can be diagnosed before pregnancy and also in early pregnancy. The cervical stitch is a surgical procedure done around the 14th week of pregnancy with a success rate of roughly 85%–90%. It is important that congenital malformations of the uterus be ruled out, preferably before pregnancy. Sometimes these malformations coexist with an incompetent cervix. If such a malformation exists, then it may be corrected surgically (depending upon the malformation).

If you are suffering from hypertension, you need to be investigated thoroughly before the next pregnancy to find out the possible cause, and see that the blood pressure is under control before attempting the next pregnancy. I could not figure out the need to give you hCG (Profasi) injections.

153. What should I do for my high-risk pregnancy?

Q. I had to terminate my first pregnancy in the 11th week last year because the baby was suffering from anencephaly. Now I am pregnant again and it is my 12th week. I had a 3-D scanning in my 11th week and the report was normal. I am taking 5 mg folic acid every day. Do I still have a high-risk pregnancy? I also underwent laparoscopic surgery 2 months ago. During that time I conceived but didn't know about it. The doctor says that everything is fine. Please advise.

A. The term 'high-risk pregnancy' is a technical term used by doctors to categorize the kind of care that a patient requires in pregnancy. It includes tests and check-ups that are additionally done compared with those used in low- or normal-risk pregnancies, to ensure a happy outcome. It does not imply that there is anything wrong with this pregnancy. It just reminds the doctor and the medical team that you need extra special care.

Once the additional blood tests and ultrasound scans are done from now up to the 5th month and are normal, you will be reclassified as a 'precious pregnancy'.

A good 3-D ultrasound scan between 11 and 14 weeks is adequate to exclude anencephaly. A follow-up scan is required at 18–20 weeks to exclude other structural abnormalities. Your doctor has already confirmed the absence of risk from anaesthesia during laparoscopy. Relax and enjoy your pregnancy!

154. Is a high amniotic volume index (AVI) dangerous for the fetus?

Q. I am 26 weeks pregnant. Recently, I underwent an ultrasound out of self-interest. Everything was normal but the amniotic volume index (AVI) value was 18. I got some sugar tests done around 2 months back as I had an

operation for an abscess in the back. But the results were normal. My parents were diabetic and are no more now. The doctor has advised for some sugar-related tests. I have already had 3 miscarriages in the first trimester and this is a precious baby for me. How serious is this and what complications can it create? What medications and personal precautions should I take to reduce this value?

A. The normal amniotic fluid index (AFI), also known as amniotic volume index (AVI), is 12–14 cm. The reading of 18 indicates a mild increase. The causes of this are several and include high blood sugar, fetal malformations and infections. The vast majority of patients with a high AVI do not have any specific cause. A careful ultrasound scan can exclude most (but not all) malformations. Blood tests on the mother are useful to exclude specific infections. Raised blood sugar levels are a common cause. These can by assessed be simple blood tests. Once these sinister causes have been excluded, the fluid needs to be monitored frequently and a premature rupture of the water bag needs to be prevented by restricting your activity and treating the underlying cause if discovered. By itself this is not a problem to be alarmed about.

155. How is oligohydramnios managed?

Q. My wife is 24 years old, pregnant and suffering from oligohydramnios. She does not have diabetes or hypertension. She is 26 weeks pregnant. The doctor said that the growth of the baby is lagging by two weeks. How should this be managed? She has been taking IV amino acids. How much of this should be taken and at what duration? Please advise.

A. Oligoamnios or oligohydramnios, or reduced fluid around the unborn baby has several causes. An ultrasound can exclude abnormalities of the fetal urinary tract as a possible cause. Additionally, colour Doppler studies with the ultrasound can detect poor placental function or reduced flow through the mother's uterine blood vessels. If these factors are excluded, the treatment lies in adequate maternal fluid intake, plenty of rest, a good diet and medication with progesterone. Intravenous drips have not conclusively been proven to be useful. The same treatment will also improve the growth of the baby. Trips to the doctor and ultrasound scans will need to be more frequent and delivery may be required before the due date.

Congenital malformations in the baby, placental insufficiency, and preterm leakage need to be ruled out. Amnioinfusion (injecting fluid into the uterus, around the baby) is another management option, which is useful in preventing limb reduction defects (amputation of the limbs caused by adhesions), and pulmonary hypoplasia (underdevelopment of the lungs). Amnioinfusion should to be done by an experienced perinatologist. Your wife should have antenatal care in a tertiary centre with good neonatal ICU facilities.

156. What happens if there is less fluid in the mother's womb?

Q. My wife is pregnant and in the 28th week. Now the doctor has informed us after sonography that the baby's growth is not adequate and its weight is less than normal. Even the growth of some crucial parts like the brain is less than normal. He has advised her to take bed rest from now on. He also said that the fluid in the mother's womb is less than normal. Now he has asked for a weekly check-up. None of the above was pointed out in earlier check-ups. This is our first baby and we wish to have no problems for both the baby and the mother.

A. This condition, where the fluid in the mother's womb is less, is called oligohydramnios, whereby the baby has less space to move. This can manifest late during pregnancy. You need weekly check-ups by your gynaecologist/obstetrician. Your wife should maintain a daily fetal kick count. A colour Doppler study can be helpful. Blood pressure should be checked every week. A malformation scan should be repeated. You should deliver in a good hospital with a good neonatal care unit so that, if the baby's birth weight is low, it can be well looked after.

157. Is it dangerous to deliver a baby in the 8th month?

Q. I am 30 years old and in my 8th month of pregnancy. In the first week of the 8th month, the doctor did a scan and told me that the baby is very low and his head is almost down. He advised bed rest and asked me not to move till I finish the 8th month. Is it dangerous to deliver the baby in the 8th month? Will resting all the time without moving help me go through my 8th month without delivering?

A. It is best if the baby delivers at term (37 completed weeks of pregnancy). If the baby is born at the end of the 8th month, it is not very 'bad' because you will be 35 weeks by then. However, a preterm baby may have to face many problems, including breathing and feeding problems as well as difficulty in maintaining the body temperature.

If your doctor has advised rest, I agree with her. Bed rest does help in prolonging pregnancy. It is best to have the delivery as close to term as possible, and preferably at term.

158. How safe is it to conceive after 35 years of age?

Q. I am 36 years old. My older child is 7 years old. Can I go in for another baby at this age?

A. Generally speaking, fertility in women declines with advancing age. After the age of 35, certain adverse pregnancy outcomes do occur in pregnant women. These include gestational diabetes, pregnancy-induced hypertension (PIH), antepartum haemorrhage (bleeding during pregnancy after 28 weeks), labour disorders and a higher risk of chromosomal anomalies in the baby. The increased rates of preterm labour and caesarean section in women above 35 years are probably due to the increased incidence of medical disorders noted in these women.

All that said, we all know of healthy children born to women in their late 30s and 40s. I would strongly recommend that you see a fertility specialist, and get a thorough evaluation of your hormone levels, your ovulation, and some education on your fertile period.

159. Can I conceive at the age of 39?

Q. I am 39 years old with a 7-year-old girl. Since last year, I have high blood pressure and have been taking medication (telmisartan 20 mg). When there is tension at home, my BP rises to 180/120 mmHg. Under such conditions, can I conceive? Will the pregnancy period be safe? Will the baby be normal?

A. All pregnancies in women over the age of 36 years are considered risky. This is irrespective of the blood pressure, whether normal or not.

Use of Telmisartan during pregnancy is not permitted since the baby's exposure to this drug can cause both fetal and neonatal morbidity, serious and severe malformation, and even death. Telmisartan is also not allowed during breastfeeding. You should very carefully think whether it is worth trying to conceive. In the meantime, please use effective contraception so that even by mistake you do not become pregnant because of the inherent danger to the fetus.

160. Is pregnancy possible at the age of 50?

Q. I am 50 years old. I got married very late and now I want to get pregnant. My monthly periods have stopped. I have no disease and I am a healthy and strong woman, working as a teacher. Science has advanced so much that everything is possible nowadays. Is there any way for me to get pregnant indirectly, by sperm, egg, or ovary donation? Please advise.

A. To achieve a successful pregnancy after menopause with ART, using donor egg, is even more complicated and expensive as compared with ART with donor egg before the menopause. In this case, I would strongly recommend that you adopt a baby, as that would give an orphan a home and love, and satisfy your maternal instincts. You would, however, have to check whether or not adoption is permitted at this age. Another point to note is that having a baby at this age (whether by ART or through adoption) is not easy, as tolerance levels go down with advancing age. Also, the baby would not reach adulthood by the time the woman becomes a senior citizen, which is not fair for the child.

Problems of the fetus

161. Why have the fetal movements decreased during pregnancy?

Q. I am 9 months pregnant. For the past 2 weeks the movements of the baby have become very few (compared to 5–7 months). The doctor did get the routine scan done and everything seems to be normal. Please tell me if it is normal for the number of movements to come down at this stage. What should be the number of movements per hour, so that I can keep a count? My hands and legs have started swelling (anklets and rings are getting tight!). During the previous 8 months there was no swelling. My blood pressure has continued to be normal throughout. Is there anything to worry about?

A. The mother's count of the baby's movements (fetal kick count) is a very good indicator of fetal well-being. There should be at least 12 strong movements in a day (from the time the woman wakes up in the morning till the evening, i.e. 5 p.m.). If the movements are 'weak', less than 12, or less than 50% of the usual kick count, the woman should report this immediately to the obstetrician, who will definitely assess the fetal condition and decide what to do. After 35 weeks, one need not be too worried about delivering the baby.

162. Will a transverse lie position of the fetus lead to any complications?

Q. I am 5 months and 2 weeks pregnant. On anomaly scan, it was found that my baby is in a transverse lie. What are the chances of the baby

changing its position by the time of delivery? If the baby doesn't change its position, will it affect its development in any way? I want to avoid caesarean section. Could you please suggest any methods that I can adopt to change the position of my baby?

A. Until late in pregnancy, which means 30–40 weeks, the fetus floats free in the uterus. It has no fixed position. The position fixes only in the last 3 weeks. Therefore, it is perfectly normal to have a baby in a transverse lie at your stage of pregnancy. The baby will take up a position on its own later and there is nothing that needs to be done to ensure a normal final position. That is Nature's job and does not need any help from you! The position of the baby does not affect its development.

If the baby is noted to be in a transverse lie after 32 weeks of pregnancy, certain conditions that predispose to it should be ruled out. These are: malformations in the shape of the uterus, placenta praevia, a tumour in the lower part of uterus (e.g. fibroid) or pelvis, and a pendulous abdomen of the mother (e.g. a woman with 5 children who has lax abdominal wall muscles).

163. What is the importance of femur length during pregnancy?

Q. Is it possible to know from an ultrasound of an 8-month fetus whether the child is going to be short or tall in height after birth? What is the role of femur bone in this respect? What steps can be taken in case the child is short? Is there any special technique or medicine for proper growth and to increase the height, assuming that all care is taken during pregnancy? Please advise.

A. Femur length or the length of the thigh bone is an index of fetal growth in the uterus. This can be measured during an ultrasound examination. In the last three months of pregnancy, the longer the bone, the longer is the length of the baby at birth. However, it is not an index of the final growth of the adult. A good nutritious diet and adequate amounts of rest and sleep are enough to achieve the growth potential of the unborn child. In a few cases, extra care may be required. Your obstetrician would be the best person to decide on these factors. No medication can enhance the height.

164. Why is the femur of my fetus short?

Q. My pregnancy corresponds to 27–31 weeks. The details of the USG report are: BPD – 76, FL – 51, abdominal circumference – 239, head circumference – 261 and the fetal weight – 1.2 kg. The doctor says that the femur length seems to be small. Is it something to worry about? I am 4 feet 11 inches tall and my husband's height is 5 feet 4 inches. Please advise.

A. The head size and abdominal perimeter in this report correspond to 27–28 weeks' size. The length of the femur is also within the normal range for this period, but is on the lower side of the normal range. This is expected when the parents are both in a similar height range, as in this case. If you want to be doubly sure that this is a normal variant and not a disorder of bone growth and development, it would be wise to do a repeat ultrasound scan which includes an assessment of the length of all bones of all limbs and also assess the overall architecture of the bones. This would confirm a normal variant and exclude a skeletal disorder.

165. Why am I not feeling any fetal movements?

Q. I am 5 months pregnant. I had an ultrasound done during my 18th week. Everything was normal except that the movements were less. The doctor said that I could fly to US. I haven't experienced any movement as yet. I had a missed abortion last time. I weighed 60 kg in my first month and weigh 64 kg now. I am fully fit and don't feel that I am pregnant. I don't feel tired. I just want to make sure that my baby and I are all right. I took 4 doses of hCG injection. I am now taking iron, folic acid and calcium tablets. Please relieve me of my tension.

A. Each pregnancy holds different experiences for the mother and what is a general rule in pregnancies is not the rule for each one of them. This is the essence of biology and medicine. There is a very wide range of normal events. Since a scan at 18 weeks and your check-up with your doctor were normal, it is likely that all is well. Actual kicking is felt later in pregnancy. Since this is the first pregnancy where you have reached the fifth month or 20 weeks, you may or may not have realized that organized gas and flutters are actually movements of the baby. In your next visit to your doctor in the US you will get to hear the heart beat of your baby and feel reassured. Your doctor is also likely to get the 20-week scan carried out which is done anytime between 18 and 22 weeks. It is natural to be anxious if one has had a previous miscarriage, as in your case. Relax as much as you can and enjoy your new surroundings and the pregnancy.

166. What complications can arise if the cord is around the neck of the baby?

Q. I am 35 weeks pregnant. My ultrasound report says that 2 loops of cord are seen in the region of the nape of the neck – one a stradle and one around. What complications can this lead to? My first child was born by a caesarean section.

A. The cord is around the neck in 27 out of every 100 babies who have an ultrasound in the last month of pregnancy. Most of these are of no consequence. Occasionally (in about 1 of these 100 babies) the cord tightens around the neck during labour and then the baby gets choked. This may result in death or mental disability of the baby. Therefore, when this observation is made in an ultrasound scan, the obstetrician monitors the baby's heart beat during labour, as a distressed baby will first show an increase in heart rate and then a fall. Whenever there is a doubt regarding the baby's safety as reflected in the heart rate pattern, an emergency caesarean section can be performed. If the heart rate remains steady, a normal delivery is carried out. Please also note that the cord can come off the neck even before labour begins and then of course there is absolutely no problem.

A repeat ultrasound colour Doppler scan is recommended at the start of labour, at 40 weeks, or before terminating the pregnancy. If this confirms the condition has not changed, caesarean section should be performed.

167. What is the reason for the absence of heartbeat in the fetus?

Q. I am a 30-year-old housewife, residing in Saudi Arabia. My son is 3 years 3 months old. I have been suffering from excessive bleeding during menstruation for which the doctor prescribed Marvelon tablets for 6 months. There was some improvement. I also suffered from migraine and was prescribed Inderal tablets, which I took for almost 2 months. When we visited India, I consulted a doctor who prescribed Sibelium 0.5 mg once daily. As my headaches stopped, I discontinued the medicine. I had also been suffering

from stress/tension earlier and had taken medication for the same, which I discontinued a year ago. I had regular menstrual periods with a 28-day cycle. My last menstrual period was 3 months ago. My pregnancy test done last month was positive. I was prescribed folic acid tablets on my first visit. The result of the ultrasound scan showed a fetus about 5–6 weeks of age. I underwent one more ultrasound scan after which the doctor told me that the heartbeat of the fetus could not be heard and there was no growth. I was told that the fetus might come out at any time. If there was no bleeding, I was advised to visit the doctor again to remove it. What is the cause of death of the fetus? Could food poisoning have harmed it? When can I get pregnant again?

A. Most early abortions are because of what is called an anembryonic pregnancy, meaning that the fetus is never really formed. This is because of an abnormality in the fetus and is an accident of nature. In any given semen specimen, about 30% sperm are abnormal and by the same logic many eggs are abnormal as well. When an abnormal sperm or egg mates, there is an abnormal fetus. This aborts and it is best that it aborts rather than develops into an abnormal baby. Almost 50% of all early pregnancies abort (about 20% after a diagnosis and others even earlier). Reproductive wastage is an unavoidable event in nature. Since you already have a normal child there is nothing to worry about. Once the diagnosis is confirmed by a good ultrasound examination, you should abort this pregnancy. You do not have to wait at all before you plan another one (the traditional advice of waiting for six months has no proven scientific rationale). Please do not worry – there is no defect.

There are no precautions or drugs with which we can prevent these early abortions and even if we could, we should not as it would lead to abnormal babies. This is natural selection (Darwinism) and we should not interfere with it. You do not need any tests or precautions and no medicines except folic acid in the next pregnancy also. Meanwhile, if the diagnosis is confirmed, please get a medical/surgical termination done.

168. Can the breech position of the baby lead to symphysis pubis dysfunction in the mother?

Q. I am 30 weeks pregnant and suffer from symphysis pubis dysfunction. I had a scan and the baby is in the breech position. Is this making my pain worse? Is there enough room for the baby to change its position on its own without help?

A. Pregnancy does cause some tolerable pain in the bones of the pelvis and spine. If you already have some problem with the symphysis pubis, the pain is sure to get aggravated with advancing pregnancy. Regarding the baby changing his position (which normally occurs after the 32nd week), there are many causes for persistent breech presentation – one of them is a contracted pelvis. It is not possible to predict what will happen in your case without a physical examination.

169. What is the reason for non-detection of the fetal stomach in my case?

Q. I am 22 years old. I have now had 7 anomaly scans and I am 27 weeks pregnant. The doctor has still not been able to find the fetal stomach. Nobody seems to be explaining the reason to me. I have been told that there is a problem and my baby will undergo surgery when he is born and that I will have to deliver in a hospital with a special care unit. However, they are still unforthcoming with details saying that I have to wait for an appointment with another consultant. I understand that this is a hard case to comment on, but I want more information on this. Where should I go for information? If I know what the possible problems might be, at least I will be able to prepare myself better. Please advise.

A. Failure to visualize the fetal stomach on repeated scanning indicates that the stomach does not fill or is not in the normal location. If it is not in its normal location then it is usually in the chest where it can be located with a careful ultrasound. The other causes of non-filling are problems of swallowing such as cleft lip and palate, brain abnormalities, failure of formation of the foodpipe and lumps in the baby's neck. Many of these can be assessed on a careful ultrasound and with 3-D/4-D ultrasound. The outlook depends on the cause and its surgical correctibility and on associated abnormalities. Often, the condition is associated with increased amounts of fluid surrounding the baby and this may predispose to a premature delivery. Prematurity has a negative influence on the final outcome. A fetal medicine specialist and a paediatric surgeon may give more information after studying the reports.

Placental abnormalities

170. Do blood clots in the placenta harm the fetus?

Q. Do blood clots in the placenta cause any deformity in the fetus? What are the causes of blood clotting during pregnancy? How can we avoid this in the next pregnancy? What safety measures can be taken?

A. A huge blood clot can lead to placental insufficiency and growth restriction of the baby, and even death of the fetus at times. Tiny blood clots can also cause placental insufficiency and growth restriction but as such they do not result in fetal malformations.

There are many causes of small blood clots in the placental vessels, resulting in placental insufficiency. The commoner ones are pregnancy-induced hypertension (PIH), essential hypertension, diabetes mellitus and antiphospholipid antibody syndrome in the mother. These have to be ruled out and treated, if present. Before the next pregnancy, please take the following precautions: (i) Rule out these medical disorders; (ii) get treated, if you are diagnosed with any such disease before attempting the next pregnancy; (iii) good antenatal care is a must to detect PIH early.

171. Will a low-lying placenta harm my pregnancy?

Q. I am 13 weeks pregnant. The ultrasound detected a low-lying placenta. What precautions do I need to take?

A. Vaginal intercourse, heavy work and travelling on bumpy roads should be avoided. However, most of the low placentas migrate up as the pregnancy advances. You should report to the nearest hospital or your doctor at the onset of slightest bleeding (even spotting).

172. What does a grade 3 placenta mean?

Q. My wife is pregnant and one week short of entering the 8th month. The doctor did an ultrasound scanning and said that she suspects my wife's placenta to be in grade 3 of early stage. She asked us to go for a Doppler scan. What does this mean? How will it affect her delivery?

A. A grade 3 placenta indicates calcification within the placenta. This usually occurs after 35 weeks or in those with placental insufficiency. It is definitely a point of concern if present at 30 weeks, even in the absence of hypertension and diabetes. A colour Doppler of the mother's uterine arteries and of the umbilical cord of the baby will give a good idea of the degree of placental insufficiency and fetal well-being. Your wife will need intensive monitoring, and may require preterm delivery of the baby.

173. What is the reason for premature placental ageing?

Q. My wife has completed 30 weeks and 4 days of gestation. She underwent an ultrasound scan and the doctor said that it was a case of premature placenta (grade 3 in the 31st week). The baby's weight is 1.5 kg and it measures 16 inches from head to toe. Her blood pressure was 120/80 mmHg (normal). Can premature placenta lead to complications?

A. Premature ageing (grade 3) of the placenta can occur in conditions such as pregnancy-induced hypertension, diabetes mellitus, and can be associated with intrauterine growth retardation (IUGR, small for date baby) and placental insufficiency leading to chronic fetal distress. I suggest you ensure the scan has been done by an experienced sonologist. The findings have to be correlated with the clinical findings. Discuss this scan report with your gynaecologist/obstetrician, and she will guide you as to what to do next – in terms of treatment and further tests. It is best not to do a self-diagnosis – since it can lead to unnecessary confusion and stress.

174. Is my ultrasound report of the placenta normal?

Q. How are the placental grades in pregnancy interpreted? Is it normal to have a placenta-fundal posterior grade 0 at 13 weeks of pregnancy?

A. This report of the placenta is absolutely normal. I guess your baby's heartbeats and growth have been documented to be normal by an ultrasound. Grading of the placenta depends upon the sonographic morphology, with grade 3 indicating a mature placenta, usually at term.

Appendix

I. Diet during pregnancy
II. Pregnancy after 35
III. Exercises during pregnancy
IV. Resources

Diet during pregnancy*

Q. When a woman gets pregnant, does she have to eat for two people?

A. Eating in pregnancy depends on the weight in the beginning. In the first trimester one does not need extra calories *per se*, but one needs to have lots of vitamins and folic acid because all tissues are growing and the fetus is beginning to form, so vitamins and minerals are most essential and of course proteins. As the trimester progresses, one must start eating extra in terms of proteins because the body is growing inside. You need lots of milk or milk products and whole grains. Healthy eating is very important during pregnancy, you must eat a healthy normal diet.

Q. Why has diet become such a big issue nowadays?

A. Now it is a matter of survival of the fittest. The intelligence of a child depends a lot on the diet the mother has during pregnancy. Most educated girls are positive about these contributions; that is why they like to eat the right type of diet before and during pregnancy.

Q. Most women end up gaining a lot of weight when they are pregnant, and once the baby is delivered the weight is still intact. Why does this happen?

A. They generally go wrong at the beginning because they eat food that is rich in calories, for example, we recommend a lot of low-fat milk but they end up taking high-fat milk. There is a lot of pressure on using *ghee* in the diet especially in north India. People usually take a lot of *ghee* in their diet. So, if you take too much of refined and dense foods in terms of fats and sugars, of course you will gain weight. You have to eat satiety

* Based on the transcript of a live Q&A programme telecast on NDTV 24X7

food that stays in the stomach for a long time and not refined food. This way you do not gain too much weight.

Q. When does the food craving in pregnancy start? Can this be the cause for the excessive weight gain?

A. In the first trimester it is very common to have these cravings and I don't think we should stop them as long as women take hygienic food and eat whatever they feel like. Subsequently, if we find that they are going overboard and gaining too much weight, we advise them, which is usually during the second trimester and much more in the third.

Q. Would you say that doctors nowadays tell women not to eat too much instead of eating?

A. Yes, we have to tell them that because most of them eat things which we would not want them to eat. But in the first trimester we do not worry about this.

Q. I am anaemic and right now my haemoglobin count is 10.1. We are planning a child but we don't know what I should eat, because no matter what I eat my haemoglobin count does not go above 10.1.

A. A haemoglobin of count of 10.1 g/dl is not too bad by Indian standards, so you should not worry. You should first analyse if there is any other cause for the anaemia. We must exclude the possibility of your carrying a thalassaemic trait. Once that is clear you can concentrate on your diet. Take a high protein, high iron-containing diet and may be some supplement of vitamins. Also take folic acid right from now.

Q. What is the role of folic acid in pregnancy?

A. These days we recommend the intake of folic acid even during the pre-pregnancy stage, i.e. when the person is planning a pregnancy. It is good to take folic acid because there is documented proof that the outcome of the fetus is much better in women who take folic acid during pregnancy.

Q. I am in the 3rd month of my pregnancy, what food should I eat to relieve constipation?

A. You need to take a lot of fibre in your diet. First of all when you eat breakfast, you should not take white bread, either take whole wheat bread or porridge or oats. During lunch and dinner, you should take whole wheat gram or whole wheat flour. You can mix some soybeans or Bengal gram flour in the wheat. You should take plenty of fruits and vegetables. Drink lots of fluids too. Refined carbohydrates should be avoided and more roughage should be added to the diet.

Q. What exercises should a 3-month pregnant lady do?

A. She should walk to maintain her physical activity to the maximum.

Q. My wife is pregnant and feels very hungry. What kind of food should I give her?

A. This is very normal and she will feel hungry as the baby keeps growing. She needs to take a lot of proteins in her diet. She should take at least 2 glasses of milk and 2 bowls of pulses and lots of soybean. She should not take too much hollow calories such as sugar and fats. Hunger is normal but foods that are high in protein and roughage will curtail the hunger and she will not gain extra weight.

Q. Is it advisable to eat smaller meals?

A. It is more satisfying especially if you are not working and are at home. Then you can take a small breakfast at 11 a.m. and then take your lunch. It is much better to have smaller meals but try to curtail the amount of fat and sugar.

Q. I am pregnant for the past 5 months and am carrying twins. What should be my diet and how much weight do I need to put on? The doctor says it is between 11 and 14 kg for a normal child but I am carrying twins so will it be more than 14 kg?

A. The aim should be to put on 1–2 kg in a month. You must eat at short intervals and in small amounts. Don't eat too much because if you do you will feel uncomfortable. So, eat nutritious food at short intervals, and cut down on your fat and sugar intake.

Q. I am 2 months pregnant and I suffer from polio in my left leg since I was 10 months old. I want to know whether I have to be more careful about my diet and what precautions I should take during pregnancy.

A. You don't have to worry about your polio as of now. You are just like any other pregnant girl, so eat whatever your doctor advises. You have to avoid excess weight gain and subsequently when you are near term, then your doctor will decide whether your pelvis is adequate for a normal delivery and that is the only difference. Otherwise, there is no difference.

Q. I am 4 months pregnant and I have heartburn. How can I avoid this?

A. Heartburn is common in early pregnancy. You should avoid taking too many spices. You should not remain on an empty stomach for too long, take small frequent meals and avoid deep-fried food. Whenever you are hungry, take cold milk or something that will neutralize the acid.

Q. What should women suffering from diabetes and hypertension do during pregnancy?

A. In the beginning they have to be very conscious. The factors that contribute to the exacerbation of these symptoms of hypertension or diabetes must be curbed right from the beginning. In the diet, they have to be careful of reducing the intake of salt and sugar. They must have frequent check-ups to keep a check on the blood pressure and diabetes, and if detected they should be treated by diet or medication.

Q. I am 8 months pregnant. Is there any special diet I should take?

A. You should take a balanced diet that includes a lot of proteins. You should take two to three glasses of milk and if you don't like milk you can take *paneer* or curd. You should continue with whatever exercise allowed to you by your doctor.

Q. What are the harmful effects of eating too many carbohydrates in pregnancy?

A. When there is an excess intake of carbohydrates, there is excessive weight gain which is not desirable. The woman feels bloated and some may develop gas problems too.

Q. My wife is 7 months pregnant and wants to have food containing garlic and ginger. Should she be allowed to have it?

A. There is no harm in having garlic and ginger but she should try to avoid too much of fried food.

Q. I am 11 weeks pregnant and weigh 35 kilos. Can I eat dry fruits?

A. Yes, you can take dry fruits, especially almonds.

Pregnancy after 35*

Q. Are pregnancies after 35 becoming more common nowadays?

A. Yes, nowadays pregnancies after 35 are quite common, especially since the last decade. This is common not only in developed countries but also in our clinics, and we see patients who are 35, 36 and even 40 years olds, who come to ask whether they are pregnant or not. It is because of the change in lifestyle. Women are active in all fronts and that is why they delay pregnancy.

Q. What are the risks involved in pregnancy after 35?

A. The risk starts right from the time of conception. The infertility rate is much higher after the age of 35. Once a 35-year-old woman becomes pregnant, the risk of miscarriage is much higher. There is a 20% risk of miscarriage at 35. There is a higher risk of abnormalities, particularly Down syndrome, in the child. Then there are the risks of premature labour, and of hypertension and diabetes in late pregnancy. Labour is difficult and they have a higher caesarean section rate. At every stage the child and the mother will encounter problems if the woman is above 35 years.

Q. What are the positive results of having children after 35?

A. There are couple of things that are good about an older mother. She is much more confident. She is usually financially independent. She can provide better for her child. Children of older mothers are known to do better in schools. These parents are more likely to stay together. Older parents are more stable and caring, thus their children do better.

---

* Based on the transcript of a live Q&A programme telecast on NDTV 24X7

Q. What is Down syndrome?

A. The exact cause of Down syndrome is not known. As the woman grows older her eggs also tend to get older. When these eggs are fertilized, the combination results in an extra chromosome, which causes Down syndrome. The child born with an extra chromosome may be handicapped or have a low IQ.

Q. Why do older women need to control their sugar when planning a pregnancy?

A. Older women are more likely to have pre-existing diabetes and hypertension. If they don't have it preconceptionally, then in the course of the pregnancy they are prone to develop gestational diabetes as well as pregnancy-induced hypertension. Diabetes in pregnancy can be very traumatic for both the mother and the child.

Q. What precautions does an already diabetic woman need when she's planning a pregnancy?

A. In such cases you have to be very careful right from the beginning. You cannot be on oral antidiabetic drugs. You have to be on insulin. You have to keep a very strict control on the diabetes. If you do, you will do reasonably well like any other normal woman. Uncontrolled blood sugar levels can cause unexplained fetal death. This is a high-risk pregnancy and should be managed in a well-equipped hospital.

Q. Most of the post-35 pregnancies are planned. Hence women have enough time to prepare for them. What precautions can they take beforehand to avoid problems later?

A. Older women planning a pregnancy must see an obstetrician and gynaecologist beforehand. The doctor should take a detailed history of the couple to find out if there is any history of malformation in the family. Second, if there is any history of diabetes, then the doctor should investigate the couple thoroughly, especially the woman. If the woman is obese, she should regulate her weight. If she is diabetic then the drug has to be changed when she is planning a pregnancy. If she is hypertensive her blood pressure has to be controlled.

Q. Does the age of the man affect a normal delivery?

A. Men are lucky because their age is not as significant as that of women, since women contribute the egg. Unless there is an abnormality due to old age or an abnormal sperm, a genetic defect cannot be transmitted from the father to the child. But once the child is formed and is normal there is no contribution from the man.

Q. I am 38 years old and I am overweight by 25 kg. I have a 7-year-old child and I am hypertensive. How safe is it for me to have a pregnancy at this stage?

A. You are already in a high-risk category. You are overweight and hypertensive. You have to be very careful right from the beginning. You have to watch your weight. You can't lose much weight in pregnancy but it is all right if an overweight person stays at the same weight. If you are careful through your pregnancy and you have a hospital delivery, then you should do reasonably well. It is safer for a woman today to have a pregnancy at this age than it used to be earlier.

Q. What should be the ideal weight before pregnancy so that there are no problems if one puts on some weight when planning a pregnancy?

A. The optimum weight depends upon the age and the height of the patient. We have to calculate the body mass index of the patient. We try and control the patient's weight. During pregnancy, patients who are on the higher side gain less weight as compared to patients who are well maintained. We advise these patients to avoid fried foods and take exercise.

Q. Is it true that fertility rates go down after 25 in Indian women? What are the best options to conceive naturally in women beyond 35? Which dates are better during a woman's cycle? What are the artificial ways of conception?

A. Fertility does go down after the age of 25. Regarding the best days for natural conception – it depends on the length of the menstrual cycle. If a patient has a menstrual cycle of 28–30 days, the best days for the patient to conceive would be anywhere from day 12 to day 16. If she has a shorter cycle then in that case the best days would range from day 10 to day 15. Obese patients may have a cycle that ranges up to 45 days; in that case we do an ultrasound to find out when they are ovulating. Intrauterine insemination (IUI), guided by cycle monitoring, is one of the artificial ways of conception without giving drugs. This method increases ovulation induction and the patient is made to conceive. We can also do *in vitro* fertilization (IVF).

Q. Are there any tests to detect abnormalities in the child during the early stages of pregnancy?

A. Definitely, now the focus is more on early diagnosis because it is less traumatic for the parents if the problem is diagnosed earlier. In the first trimester, there is a test for Down syndrome – a sonography test for nuchal translucency. We measure the thickness of the skin fold behind the neck of the baby. These are very sensitive tests, which pick up abnormalities in the child, particularly for Down syndrome. New combined blood tests are also being introduced, which can be performed in the first and second trimester.

There are the triple marker and quadruple marker tests, which are very indicative, especially of Down syndrome. There is a three-dimensional sonography test where one can see the baby almost like it would be seen outside the womb. One can investigate every small part of the baby to look for abnormalities.

Q. My wife is above 35 and she is on medication for epilepsy. We have 2 children, but we want to go for a third one. Can we proceed?

A. First of all, you must consult a neurologist to know if the epilepsy is well controlled. Second, your wife should switch to a drug that is safe during pregnancy. Third, she should start taking folic acid. She is 35 years old and has two children. If you want to have more children, you can surely plan a pregnancy. It would be better to undergo a blood test and ultrasound before deciding.

Q. The risks of pregnancy start from the age of 35 – what about 33 and 34?

A. The age of 35 is not a well-defined limit. For example, if we take the example of Down syndrome, there is a risk of Down syndrome at the age of 25 but it is 1 in 1250. At 35, the risk is 1 in 385. The risk increases with age. It is not that the risk does not exist at a younger age. Similarly, a lady in the younger age group can develop hypertension during pregnancy, she can develop diabetes too, she may have a growth-retarded baby and she may end up with a caesarean section. The same things can happen at a young age, it is just that the chances of them happening at an older age are more.

Q. I am 40 years old; can I go for IVF at this age?

A. Sure, you can go ahead for IVF.

Exercises during pregnancy*

Q. Many women go through a dilemma of whether or not to exercise during pregnancy. They are told by elders not to exercise. What do you suggest?

A. Yes, this is a common belief we have in India, probably from the fact that women did a lot of physical work earlier, they milked the cows and worked in the fields, but in the urban setting a woman does need to exercise since it helps her in various ways. It prepares her body for a natural delivery, it keeps her body supple and flexible and is good for her general well-being.

Q. Why are women advised to exercise? Does it help in having an easier delivery, and does it make them lose weight faster after the delivery?

A. Yes, the muscle tone is regained faster after they have a baby. It also prepares their body for a natural delivery.

Q. Very often doctors advise pregnant women that the first trimester of their pregnancy is very crucial, why is this?

A. The maximum number of miscarriages take place in the first trimester. If they exercise and happen to bleed coincidently, then the patient gets very upset. It is important to be very careful during the first trimester.

Q. For how long during pregnancy is one allowed to exercise? Can you exercise till the 9th month?

A. It really depends on the situation during pregnancy, but if you have a

* Based on the transcript of a live Q&A programme telecast on NDTV 24X7

perfectly normal pregnancy, you can exercise or do your normal activities right up to the day you go into labour.

Q. What are the common types of exercise that most women are advised?

A. I teach a mix of exercises, some of them are taken from yoga, some from physiotherapy and some from meditation. I think it is very important for a woman to be happy when she is pregnant because her thoughts influence the baby. Whatever she goes through when she is pregnant affects her child.

Q. Very often we hear about Lamaze classes being held for pregnant women, what exactly are they?

A. Lamaze is a kind of breathing technique. A doctor named Dr Ferdinand Lamaze went to Russia and learnt how the Russians taught the breathing technique and then started to teach it in France. It is a kind of breathing that is taught in antenatal classes.

Q. How does it help in the body structure?

A. Lamaze breathing doesn't help in body structure. It is totally for labour. It prepares the mother for labour and helps her to deal with the labour through breathing. Dr Lamaze felt that just like a woman learns to ride a bicycle she could learn how to handle labour through breathing.

Q. There are lot of women who usually don't exercise before pregnancy, so when they are pregnant they are especially asked to exercise. What kind of exercise would you recommend for these women?

A. I think pregnancy is the time when every woman is motivated because she wants to do her best for herself and her baby. Hence, even women who have never exercised must start during their pregnancy. The exercise does not have to be vigorous or strenuous. If a woman has never exercised before, she can do some very simple exercises such as stretching, relaxation exercises, meditation and learning deep breathing, learning to concentrate on a particular spot. These help to relieve back strain. They help you with simple problems such as varicose veins, swollen legs and constipation. Exercises relieve all these little day-to-day issues of pregnancy. But I personally feel that exercises should always be supervised. You cannot start exercising one fine day. You should start very slowly, warm up and then do about 45 minutes of exercise. Then again cool down for about 10–15 minutes. You have to take precautions such as never letting your heart rate become too fast, not more than 140 beats per minute or breathing too hard. You should always have something known as a talk test, which means you are actually able to have a conversation while exercising. If someone can actually teach you the process it is much safer.

Q. There are women who are heavily into sports; some even do heavy duty gymming before they get pregnant. Can they continue these forms of vigorous exercises during pregnancy?

A. One has to realize that in pregnancy the entire body changes. A hormone called relaxin is released, which completely relaxes the joints and ligaments. During pregnancy when you do jerky movements there is a much higher incidence of strain and sprains. Also, back strain is very common in pregnancy, as the abdomen swells up in the latter half of pregnancy and the centre of balance changes. You are much more likely to be clumsy and fall more often. You cannot do the exercises that you did earlier.

Q. My wife has been advised bed rest, can she do light exercises?

A. Anybody who has had recurrent abortions, has bleeding during pregnancy, has twins or has a low birth weight baby cannot exercise during pregnancy and is usually advised bed rest. But there is much one can do while in bed. One can do a bit of back stretching and deep breathing. One can pull the abdomen in towards the back, which will help develop a little abdominal muscle tone. One can bring your feet up and, down to strengthen the calf muscles and do pelvic floor exercises, the Kegel exercise. A lot can be done even while lying down.

Q. My wife's workplace is 12 km from our residence; can she drive during the first 3–4 months?

A. Driving should not be a problem as long as the pregnancy has been uneventful so far. Of course, the seat belt should always be in place and I hope the roads are all right.

Q. Can women who have frequent backache during pregnancy exercise?

A. Yes, in fact, exercise will help them cope better with backache.

Q. Are there any special exercises for women who suffer from backache?

A. There is something very simple that they can do. They can just go on all fours and be like that for sometime because when they are upright all the organs are wrapped in a membrane that hangs on the backbone like a flag hangs from a pole. But when she goes down on all fours then the organs hang off the back bone like clothes hang from a line and that relieves backache.

Q. Does walking help? If yes, for how long should it be done?

A. Yes, walking is very good because it gets the blood flowing. A minimum of 20–30 minutes of walking per day is good, after which the woman can put her feet up so that the blood does not pool in her legs.

Q. I am a 39-year-old ramp model. I am pregnant for the 2nd time after 2 abortions. Do I need to do anything special in terms of exercise for this?

A.Yes. Having had two abortions, you get classified as a high-risk pregnancy. As a model you need to take care of your figure and weight. I think it would be really a combination of nutrition, being careful not to put on too much weight during pregnancy, as well as some form of supervised exercise – definitely not any weight bearing. For example – not too much of brisk walking but lying on the back doing pelvic floor exercises and back-stretching exercises.

Q. What kind of exercises are suitable for pregnant women?

A. They can do butt exercises, pelvic floor exercises, exercise for the joints of the ankles, there is relaxation, shoulder rotations and lots of other exercises.

Q. Is it possible for women to continue exercises from the point of view of losing weight while they are pregnant?

A. No, pregnancy is not a time to lose weight. It is a time to maintain the abdominal tone and get a kind of aerobic effect when you walk, so that the blood flow is good.

Q. What would you advise someone who has been very conscious about weight etc. before becoming pregnant?

A. The ideal time to lose weight is pre-pregnancy but if the patient goes into pregnancy fairly overweight, the one thing we do suggest is not to put on the normal amount of weight. The normal recommendation is about 11–12 kg weight gain throughout the pregnancy. So if a woman is already overweight she can definitely put on much less – a couple of kg or sometimes even no weight gain during pregnancy. This has to be done primarily through eating a very healthy diet, being careful to cut down all excess calories; the child is very rarely deprived. The child gets its nutrition from the mother and as long as mother has a reasonable intake of calories, and supplements in terms of iron and calcium, she can provide for herself and for her baby's energy requirement without too much of caloric intake. Exercises need to be supervised and should not be overdone during pregnancy. Exercise has to be moderate and calories have to be controlled. Such a combination keeps the weight under control.

Q. Is it a myth or is it true that women cannot lose weight after giving birth to a baby?

A. It's a complete myth and women can lose weight.

Q. In the first trimester can a pregnant woman go to a hill station?

A. Normally during the first trimester, travelling should be avoided because while travelling, particularly in India, sometimes the conditions are not very comfortable. In hill stations, the roads are generally bumpy. More than anything else, in small hill stations medical facilities may not be available in case of an emergency. So, I would not recommend travelling, particularly to small towns, in the first trimester.

Resources

American College of Obstetricians and Gynecologists (ACOG)

http://www.acog.org/publications/patient_education/patientPage.cfm

The ACOG website has a section for patients, providing patient education pamphlets and health tips.

BMJ - Pregnancy

http://www.bmj.com/cgi/collection/pregnancy

The *British Medical Journal* has a section on pregnancy, providing the latest information on pregnancy.

Childbirth Connection

http://www.childbirthconnection.org

This is a non-profit organization that works to improve maternity care. The website provides information on pregnancy, labour and delivery, as well as effective pregnancy care.

Lab Tests Online – Pregnancy

http://www.labtestsonline.org/understanding/conditions/pregnancy.html

American Association of Clinical Chemistry helps patients understand clinical laboratory tests; their website has a section describing laboratory tests related to pregnancy.

MedlinePlus – Pregnancy

http://www.nlm.nih.gov/medlineplus/pregnancy.html

This site for consumers, from the US National Library of Medicine, includes information on pregnancy-related topics.

Motherisk

http://www.motherisk.org

This website, from the Hospital for Sick Children in Toronto, provides evidence-based information for consumers about the safety or risk of drugs, chemicals, and disease during pregnancy and lactation.

Royal College of Obstetricians and Gynaecologists (RCOG)

http://www.rcog.org.uk

The RCOG website has a section on information for patients with authoritative information on pregnancy-related conditions.

If you have any similar questions which need an answer, please log on to our website (http://www.DoctorNDTV.com). We have more than 290 experts on our panel and their details are accessible at our website.